PRAISE FOR

CONQUERING
CHRONIC FATIGUE

These fatigue syndromes that Dr. Forester writes about
show up all the time in my ministry. It is so refreshing to have
Christian doctors, who believe in nutrition, write on such illnesses
as these. I highly recommend this book. Get a couple of copies,
since you probably know someone who struggles with one or
more of these debilitating illnesses.

DR. NEIL T. ANDERSON
COAUTHOR, *THE BIBLICAL GUIDE TO ALTERNATIVE MEDICINE*

As I look back on my years of dealing with fibromyalgia pain
and discomfort, one of the first things that caused me great stress
and discouragement was visiting doctor after doctor and being
tested time and again only to discover from the test results that
nothing could cause my body to have this type of pain.

Dr. Forester was able to label the illness through examination
and discussion of my symptoms of pain. Under his care, I use a
combination of treatments, including medication, rest, moist heat,
exercise and the mind/body approach to healing; I have managed
to tolerate this illness and now have pain-free days.

BARBARA ATCHISON
ONE OF DR. FORESTER'S PATIENTS
LEESVILLE, LOUISIANA

Dr. Forester has clearly examined the fatigue syndromes.
He has outlined the etiologies, key symptoms, diagnosis, treatment
and prognosis of each disease. Millions of Americans who suffer from
these fatigue diseases will benefit from reading his simple yet
thorough explanations. I also liked the way Dr. Forester related the
physical etiology to spiritual etiology. He points out that our body's
health is governed by the connection of our mind, body and spirit.
Physicians as well as sufferers will benefit from reading this book.

RICHARD B. COUEY, PH.D.
PROFESSOR OF ANATOMY, PHYSIOLOGY AND NUTRITION
BAYLOR UNIVERSITY
WACO, TEXAS

Dr. Jonathan Forester has experienced success in treating
symptoms associated with chronic fatigue. His reported improvement
and remission rate is particularly impressive for those who have a
diagnosis of chronic fatigue syndrome or fibromyalgia. He examines
many other causes of chronic fatigue that may be overlooked
but can be cured with appropriate therapy. I recommend this book
to both lay and professional readers.

GEORGE A. HURST, M.D., FACP, FCCP
DIRECTOR EMERITUS, THE UNIVERSITY OF TEXAS HEALTH CENTER AT TYLER
CHAIRMAN OF THE BOARD, MINISTRY OF HEALING

In addition to the best that drug therapy can offer,
Dr. Forester adds a broad understanding of alternative
and nutritional medicine. His approach is a winning
combination that brings hope once again to those who
suffer from the perplexing fatigue syndromes.

MICHAEL D. JACOBSON, D.O.
COAUTHOR, *A BIBLICAL GUIDE TO ALTERNATIVE MEDICINE*

Conquering Chronic Fatigue appears to be a very complete study
of a challenging complex of health problems. It will require
a very thorough study, but success in treatment and recovery
for fatigue syndromes appears to be available. This book will
be an answer to many prayers.

REX RUSSELL, M.D.
INVASIVE RADIOLOGIST
AUTHOR, *WHAT THE BIBLE SAYS ABOUT HEALTHY LIVING*
WWW.BSAHEALTHYLIVING.COM

Dr. Jonathan Forester is a respected doctor and an anointed minister.
He is my personal friend and physician. He brings to this book his
medical expertise and head knowledge, along with his heart knowledge
of the God who "fearfully and wonderfully" made us all (Ps. 139:14). In
his private practice in the small southern town where we live, he has
gained a reputation for helping the helpless and healing the hopeless.
If you've ever been in a situation where the tests came back stamped
"normal"—so that you and your symptoms went home alone—you'll
want to read this book. It may just be what you need to beat fatigue!

TOMMY TENNEY
AUTHOR, *THE GOD CHASERS*

CONQUERING
CHRONIC
FATIGUE

JONATHAN
FORESTER, M.D.

Regal

From Gospel Light
Ventura, California, U.S.A.

PUBLISHED BY REGAL BOOKS
FROM GOSPEL LIGHT
VENTURA, CALIFORNIA, U.S.A.
PRINTED IN THE U.S.A.

Regal Books is a ministry of Gospel Light, an evangelical Christian publisher dedicated to serving the local church. We believe God's vision for Gospel Light is to provide church leaders with biblical, user-friendly materials that will help them evangelize, disciple and minister to children, youth and families.

It is our prayer that this Regal book will help you discover biblical truth for your own life and help you meet the needs of others. May God richly bless you.

For a free catalog of resources from Regal Books/Gospel Light, please call your Christian supplier or contact us at 1-800-4-GOSPEL *or* www.regalbooks.com.

Cover and interior design by Robert Williams
Edited by Christy Weir

Library of Congress Cataloging-in-Publication Data

Forester, Jonathan.
    Conquering chronic fatigue / Jonathan Forester.
        p.   cm.
Includes bibliographical references and index.
    ISBN 0-8307-3257-8
    1. Chronic fatigue syndrome.   2. Chronic fatigue syndrome—Religious aspects—Christianity.   I. Title.
    RB150.F37F675 2003
    616'.0478—dc21   2003010535

1   2   3   4   5   6   7   8   9   10   11   12   13   14   15   /   09   08   07   06   05   04   03

Rights for publishing this book in other languages are contracted by Gospel Light Worldwide, the international nonprofit ministry of Gospel Light. Gospel Light Worldwide also provides publishing and technical assistance to international publishers dedicated to producing Sunday School and Vacation Bible School curricula and books in the languages of the world. For additional information, visit www.gospellightworldwide.org; write to Gospel Light Worldwide, P.O. Box 3875, Ventura, CA 93006; or send an e-mail to info@gospellightworldwide.org.

DEDICATION

I dedicate this book to the Lord for His miraculous intervention
in my life, for inspiring this book and for His favor and grace.
I also dedicate this book to my best friend and wife, Cheryl;
to my four children: Brandon and his wife, Deanna, Christopher,
Andrew and Charis; to my medical office and Oasis staff; to the
men's Sunday School class; to all of my friends for their prayerful
and encouraging support; and to the countless number of
fatigued people who need a message of hope and healing.

CONTENTS

INTRODUCTION

Is the best part of your day *over* when you wake up in the morning? Or worse, when you wake up in the middle of the night and can't get back to sleep? Have you felt unusually tired day after day for months, and sleep doesn't seem to refresh you? Are you experiencing unexplained symptoms that cause you to feel weak, ill, confused and fearful? Perhaps you have seen a physician (or several) and they have given you no answers, offered little sympathy and suggested only a diagnosis of depression. In reality, you may be suffering from one of the chronic fatigue syndromes.

Maybe you've been fortunate to receive a correct diagnosis, but your physician is at a loss to help you. You look for explanations and treatment options in books and on the Internet. But you find confusing and conflicting information, and brain fog hinders your comprehension. You might be discouraged to the point where prayer seems pointless, jokes aren't funny anymore, and life has lost much of its meaning.

You are not alone. Approximately 40 million people in the United States and Canada have fatiguing illnesses. In 1992, at an American Academy of Otolaryngologic Allergy scientific meeting in Washington, D.C., Dr. Majid Ali stated that "chronic fatigue illnesses will be the scourge of the twenty-first century." Sadly, this is proving to be true. Fibromyalgia, one of the more common fatigue syndromes, is growing in epidemic proportions.

But there is hope. In the past decade, the medical community has gained an increasing understanding of the causes and effective treatments of fatigue syndromes. This book contains both traditional and natural approaches that have proven effective during the 11 years I have been treating fatigue patients. One patient in particular, Jodie, inspired me to write this book.

As a chronic fatigue syndrome (CFS) and fibromyalgia (FMS) sufferer for many years, she had been helped by neither naturopathic nor traditional practitioners. But because of a miraculous meeting and the treatments described in this book, she is in complete remission of her fatigue and pain today. The following chapter contains her story.

CHAPTER 1

THREE MEN IN AN OLD TRUCK

I call on you, O God, for you will answer me; give ear
to me and hear my prayer.

PSALM 17:6

The mountains of Colorado are a place I find respite from a somewhat stressful life, and that is where this story begins. I had been invited to spend some time at a friend's ranch and was happy for the opportunity after a busy and tiring year. I flew to Colorado Springs and then drove to the ranch near Gunnison. It was a delight to see the beautiful mountains, the purple and yellow flowers and the rapid streams where people were canoeing. As I got out of the car at the ranch, I smelled crisp, clear pine and cedar-scented air. My friends, John and Bonita Cunningham, along with a man named Ryland Robinson, met me at the door. That night I slept like a baby in the back room of the cabin where I could hear a nearby brook. I was awakened the next morning by the sounds of birds and chipmunks outside the window.

John suggested that we drive up into Gold Creek Canyon, a high mountain valley, that day. John, Ryland and I took an old Chevy truck up a gravel road to see the sights. In this pristine setting were old gold mines, aspen groves and mountains on both sides of the valley. John told me about a nearby retreat, Petra, and the woman named Jodie who ran it. We were close by, so we decided to drive by and take a look at the retreat center from the truck. Just as we were driving by, in front of the A-frame lodge, Jodie came walking down from an upper cabin to the lower part of the property where the lodge was located. We came to a stop and greeted one another, and John, who had met Jodie on a previous occasion, introduced us and mentioned that I was the president of a ministry in Louisiana called Christian Oasis (a retreat center similar to Petra). She immediately asked us to come into the lodge for a cup of coffee.

Sitting in front of a huge picture window inside the beautiful lodge, which overlooked a brook with a waterfall, I asked Jodie how often this heavenly place was used. She frowned and said, "Not very often, since I have this terrible disease." I replied, "You have fibromyalgia, don't you?" She said, "Yes," obviously wondering how I knew, having only met her a few minutes before. I told her that I had had a lot of experience with fibromyalgia and other fatigue syndromes in my practice. Jodie then described to me her 15-year history of chronic fatigue and fibromyalgia symptoms, during which neither natural approaches nor numerous visits to specialists had helped. Toward the end of our conversation, she looked at me and said, "What do you want to do with this place?" Bewildered, I asked, "What do you mean?" She said, "I want to give it to you and let you do with it what you want." "Well," I said, "we need to pray about this first!"

And so we prayed. The next day I signed a contract in which my ministry would lease the lodge and surrounding cabins for a year as an extension of Christian Oasis. Jodie then explained to me that she had planned to put this beautiful retreat center on the real estate market the next day, since she could no longer take care of it. She had been praying that if the Lord did not want her to do this, He would give her a clear sign. Three men in an old truck was her sign.

JODIE'S STORY

All my life I had been active, energetic and involved in numerous activities. As a competitive tennis player and instructor, I was in good shape. But about 15 years ago, I started feeling unusually tired after prolonged activity. Muscle pain became a constant annoyance and eventually it worsened until my muscles were continually tight and hard. They wouldn't "let go" and relax, even at night. I had other symptoms too, like burning skin, which made me feel like I was being poisoned. The fatigue was so bad for a few years that I spent most days in bed.

During these years, I saw many physicians—a general practitioner, a neurologist, a neurosurgeon and a chiropractor—to determine what was wrong with me. They tested me for lupus, MS, non-Hodgkin's lymphoma, thyroid imbalance, heart trouble, gallbladder problems and hormonal deficiencies. The test results were all normal, so I never received a diagnosis that would explain my poor heath. Without much guidance, I tried various treatments—from acupuncture to nutritional supplements to muscle-relaxing drugs. Nothing helped.

During the summers when I had a small amount of energy, my husband and I worked on building a Christian retreat center in the mountains of Colorado. We called it Petra and were blessed by the ministry it provided to groups who came to stay for a week at a time. But in 2001, I pretty much hit bottom. I was tired of smiling and trying to be sociable. I was fed up with the devastating price I had to pay for even minimal exertion. I was confused and discouraged by the continuing onslaught of odd physical symptoms that no one could explain. I was afraid that my life would never be normal again. So I prayed and told God that I would stop and do nothing and wait for Him to tell me what was wrong and what to do about it. Since I couldn't manage the retreats and the upkeep of Petra anymore, I asked the Lord to send somebody to share it, or else I was ready to put the property up for sale.

That is when I found out my younger sister had fibromyalgia. She convinced me to read a book on the condition, and there I was, right there in those miserable stories! Okay, so now I had a name for it. But what about treatment? In doing research, I found suggestions for treating the symptoms, all of them good. But I wanted to know *why* I had it and *how* to repair whatever the damage was in order to begin true healing.

On July 3, 2001, my husband and I were at Petra. I had decided that the next day we'd go into town to a realtor and explore the possibility of putting the retreat center on the market. As I was walking on the road in front of the retreat cabin, an old truck drove up. The three men in the truck inquired about the property, and I invited them to look around. As my husband and I sat down to chat with them, I mentioned I was hoping to share this place with other Christian ministries. One of the men said he was a Christian speaker and physician. He was in Colorado on vacation and had hopes of someday owning retreat property here. Then he asked me, "Do you have fibromyalgia?" I sat straight up and said, "I sure do!" He replied, "The Lord just told me that, and we're going to get you healed."

This man was Dr. Jonathan Forester from Pineville, Louisiana. Having treated many patients with fibromyalgia (FMS) and chronic fatigue syndrome (CFS), he assured me that help was available. That day Dr. Forester found the retreat he had prayed for, and I found answers and hope after suffering for over 15 years. Both our prayers were answered!

Back home in Oklahoma, I began to take the medications he prescribed and to alter my life by respecting my energy boundaries. With any chronic illness, it's easy to get stuck in a place of fear and confusion, not knowing what is happening to your body. With a proper diagnosis and effective treatments, I am now unstuck—free from pain. Instead of waking up in the morning and thinking about what is wrong with me, I wake up thinking about what God has in store for me today.

I believe my "chance" meeting with Jodie was an incredible, divine encounter! I *happened* to be in Colorado and took a sightseeing trip that just *happened* to take us near Petra. Jodie, who just *happened* to have fibromyalgia, *happened* to be walking down the hill as we drove by. We *happened* to mention our interest in a retreat center that day, 24 hours before she planned to put it up for sale. God's timing is perfect! He used our meeting to accomplish several purposes. Jodie had prayed for many years for remission from her fibromyalgia. Through the treatments I was able to offer her, she is now symptom free. She also had her prayers answered for her lovely retreat center, and my dreams of owning a place in Colorado have been fulfilled. As I write this chapter, I'm sitting in the incredible Petra lodge, thanking God for His answers to prayer and the fulfillment of His plans for us.

Be joyful in hope, patient in affliction, faithful in prayer.

ROMANS 12:12

CHAPTER 2

CAUSES OF FATIGUE

One of the most common yet undertreated and misunderstood symptoms in America is debilitating fatigue. It has been estimated that 10 to 20 percent of all Americans will experience chronic fatigue at some point in their lives. It accounts for 10 million visits a year to health-care providers. Some estimate that at least 40 million Americans and Canadians experience chronic fatigue, which is often diagnosed as depression or some other disease. Fatigue is extremely common, and I believe it will escalate due to a number of factors. These include the increasing complexity and pace of modern life, the compulsion to succeed and self-imposed demands of perfectionism. Another factor that may explain the alarming increase of fatigue

Some estimate that at least 40 million Americans and Canadians experience chronic fatigue, which is often diagnosed as depression or some other disease.

syndromes is the consumption of unhealthy foods—especially the ingestion of trans-fatty acids in cooking oils and margarine. In addition to this, the intake of high amounts of sugar, refined flours and animal fats are harmful to metabolic processes, which can contribute to fatigue syndromes. The increasing amounts of toxic chemicals in our air, water and food also put certain individuals at risk. Those with allergies are particularly sensitive to environmental toxins.

As these "stressors" bombard our bodies, they cause physical damage—especially to our central nervous system (CNS) and immune system. Add to that a lack of exercise and insufficient sleep, and it's no wonder people become not only fatigued but also are at a higher risk for depression and anxiety. Indeed, we live in a stressful world that affects our health—both emotionally and physically.

DEFINITION

Physical energy is the basis of good health. Energy is the manifestation of well-being, while fatigue is a major symptom of disease. Health is not just the absence of disease. One may think of health as the wholeness of mind, spirit and body, which provides adequate energy to meet the day's need. Some define fatigue as a sense of tiredness and lack of energy, but it must be differentiated from muscle weakness and exertional difficulties. When fatigue persists after sufficient rest from exertion, then it may be termed pathologic (disease-caused) fatigue, not simply normal fatigue.[1] Chronic fatigue is *not* caused by overexertion but is worsened by it. The following is my definition of fatigue:

> The sense of inadequate energy and malaise of mind and body, hindering one's quality of life.

The possible physiological causes of chronic fatigue can be divided into several different groupings according to the part of the body affected. Virtually any person with fatigue will have brain, immune or endocrine dysfunction.

THE BRAIN

The 100 billion-plus cells contained in the central nervous system comprise an extremely complex computer that is the master controller over all our bodily functions.[2] All chronic diseases eventually will affect neural (nervous system) processes and, therefore, one's sense of well-being. The chemicals, or neurotransmitters, that carry messages over the 10 trillion-plus brain synapses and spaces between nerve endings are integral keys to good health.[3] There probably are more than 100 different types of neurotransmitters in the brain. However, those listed below are the ones most commonly understood to play vital roles in the brain's energy system. When there is a brain-chemical imbalance, fatigue results. Later chapters will refer to these chemicals in greater detail, but here are the major ones in brief:

- Glutamate (stimulating amino acid)
- Gamma aminobutyric acid, or GABA (calming amino acid)
- Norepinephrine
- Dopamine
- Serotonin
- Histamine
- Acetylcholine

Since a large portion of the brain itself is made up of fat, adequate amounts of omega-3 essential fatty acids (EFAs) are essential to brain metabolism. Every cell in the body needs EFAs to

function, but the brain is most sensitive to a lack of this nutrient. If the brain lacks EFAs, the neural cells become stiff and less
fluid. When this occurs, vital brain chemistry is compromised;
and illnesses such as depression, anxiety, insomnia, fibromyalgia
and chronic fatigue syndrome are more likely to occur.

THE IMMUNE SYSTEM

The immune system is a set of organs that work together to rid
the body of infection. When operating correctly, the immune
system constantly attacks and destroys destructive cells and toxins without hurting the body. We only notice our immune system when it fails for some reason. For example, a cold is a sign
that your body failed to stop an antigen. (Antigens are foreign
substances such as bacteria and viruses that your body sees as
harmful invaders.) Getting over a cold is a sign that your
immune system was able to eliminate successfully the antigen.

Components of the immune system include the skin, mucous
membranes, white blood cells, bone marrow, the spleen and
lymph nodes. Their functions are listed below.

Skin
Your skin creates a physical barrier between germs and your
body. It also secretes antibacterial substances.

Mucous Membranes
The mucus in your nose and lungs contains enzymes that break
down bacteria. Saliva and tears also have antibacterial properties.

White Blood Cells
White blood cells probably are the most important part of your
immune system, because they work together to recognize and

destroy antigens (viruses, bacteria, some parasites and certain cancer cells). There are many types of white blood cells.

Bone Marrow
All cells that make up your immune system are produced in the bone marrow.

Spleen
The spleen—located in the left abdominal region near the stomach—is responsible for the destruction of red blood cells, filtration and storage of blood and production of lymphocytes.

Lymph System
Lymph nodes are found throughout your body. Your lymph vessels carry blood plasma—the clear fluid that along with the red and white blood cells constitutes your blood. Lymph nodes filter antigens from the fluid and swell up with extra white cells and dead germs when you are ill.

The immune system can malfunction in several ways. When underfunctioning, immune deficiency illnesses such as AIDS, brought on by HIV, can develop. Other diseases are the result of the immune system overreacting and attacking healthy cells. These include allergies, diabetes and autoimmune disorders such as rheumatoid arthritis, lupus and multiple sclerosis. Fatigue is one of the by-products of this immune overreaction. Important factors in healthy immune function are antioxidant nutrients, fatty acids (omega-3 oils) and regular physical activity.

THE ENDOCRINE SYSTEM
The endocrine system is composed of glands throughout the body that produce chemical messengers called hormones. The pituitary

gland, located at the base of the brain, is the master control, regulating all other glands, which include:

- Thyroid
- Adrenal
- Pineal
- Pancreas
- Ovaries
- Testicles
- Thymus

The endocrine system's chemical messengers impact every cell in your body. They affect sexual characteristics, growth, blood pressure, mineral balance, sugar metabolism, wake/sleep cycles, water retention, energy levels and many other vital activities. Recently, it has been discovered that the largest endocrine organ in your body is the endothelial cells lining the blood vessels. These 6 trillion cells—once thought to be only structural in function—are now known to liberate vital chemicals that are crucial to your well-being. If they malfunction, sludging of blood in the small capillaries can produce cholesterol buildup, causing heart attacks and strokes. We can protect the endocrine system and help keep its function in balance through adequate exercise and a healthy diet.

CELL DAMAGE AND FATIGUE

A CFS patient described her debilitating fatigue in this way:

If all the cells in my body are little power plants, I feel like they're operating at about 20 percent capacity.

The patient was correct! Each cell in your body is a tiny energy factory, and disease will almost always decrease the cell's ability to produce energy. At its basis, disease is the result of injury to the cell structure and its function. When the energy-making capacity of the body's cells has been diminished for any reason, fatigue will result. But what causes cell damage?

Cells are continually being injured and repaired. Damage can result from viral and bacterial infections; physical injury such as surgery, car accidents and burns; poor nutrition; and toxic chemicals such as environmental pollutants, food additives and drugs. Cells also are under attack by free radicals circulating through the body. A free radical is formed when a molecule loses one of its paired electrons and becomes unstable. The free-radical molecule then becomes a scavenger, attempting to steal an electron from another molecule to regain stability. Some free radicals are formed by an oxidation reaction, which is a normal process that cells use to turn food into energy. (A visible example of oxidation is a cut apple turning brown.) The free radicals naturally produced in the body are necessary for fighting infection and destroying bacteria. Only excessive free-radical production has harmful health effects. Uncontrolled free-radical formation can result from exposure to certain chemicals, radiation, cigarette smoke and other pollutants, as well as from inflammation, strenuous exercise, alcohol and a high-fat diet.

Oxidative damage to cells caused by free radicals results in a lower production of energy. Antioxidants are substances that can prevent this oxidation by supplying the missing electrons in free radicals. Using nutrients from the foods we eat, the body forms antioxidant enzymes. Consuming a diet with sufficient antioxidant nutrients is essential for cell health and energy production. Just as lemon juice, which is high in vitamin C (ascorbic acid), prevents a cut apple from turning brown, the vitamins in food can prevent oxidation in our cells. (See chapter 3 for specific antioxidant dietary recommendations.)

STRESS AND FATIGUE

One of the major causes of fatigue is excess stress. Chronic stress has a cumulative effect on every system of the body, which results in the feeling of being worn out physically and mentally. One cause is the lack of restorative sleep usually accompanying periods of stress. In addition, your adrenal glands respond to stress by producing increased levels of adrenaline, cortisol and DHEA, which are stress hormones. This adrenal response turns up bodily functions that are necessary for fight-or-flight—such as breathing, vigilance and muscle tension—and turns down nonessential responses—such as digestion and immune function. Blood is diverted into muscles; therefore, the heart races, blood pressure increases, and the skin chills. Even your spleen reacts by pumping out white blood cells, preparing for possible injury. The entire body is in a state of high alert. Your adrenal glands can become exhausted from having to operate at this peak level of efficiency over a long period of time. Whether the stress is physical (surgery or long work days) or psychological (worry, anger or relationship problems), the result is the same: an overload on your body's functions, causing fatigue. Other symptoms such as stomach problems, headaches, depression and anxiety are also ways your body attempts to get you to pay attention to the stressful aspects of your life and make appropriate changes. Stress reduction means asking yourself if a given activity recharges your batteries or depletes them. Rearranging your life's priorities through prayerful meditation, sleep, nutritional support and moderate exercise all contribute to rebuilding your adrenal health and regaining energy.

Stress reduction means asking yourself if a given activity recharges your batteries or depletes them.

CONCLUSION

Fatigue is a major symptom of a variety of illnesses and syndromes, but it is not in and of itself a disease. Finding a physician who can aggressively search for the base cause of your fatigue—rather than simply treating symptoms—is essential. Your health *will* improve as you follow the guidelines in this book, in consultation with your physician. I have treated hundreds of fatigue patients and can assure you that these treatments work.

Remember that God will guide you as you explore ways to regain your health. He will teach you and be with you in the midst of the pain, frustration and discouragement. He wants you to be well—physically, mentally and spiritually. God doesn't always heal in the ways you imagine or ask for, but He does promise to do what is ultimately best for you.

Do not fear, for I am with you; do not be dismayed, for I am your God. I will strengthen you and help you; I will uphold you with my righteous right hand.

ISAIAH 41:10

TO THE PHYSICIAN

There are several common pathways for all illnesses:

1. Virtually all diseases have an autoimmune component. This dysfunction of the immune pathway is problematic with major killers such as heart disease, stroke, cancer, lupus and fibromyalgia, among others.
2. In most illnesses, there is sludging of the blood in small capillaries as a result of dysfunction of the immune

pathway. Some health professionals propose that the blood thinner Heparin be used as therapy in illnesses such as fibromyalgia and chronic fatigue syndrome due to this sludging. It also is well known that aspirin, which is a blood thinner, helps prevent heart attacks and strokes.

3. Aging, as well as every disease, is the result of oxidant injury to some part of the cell structure and function. These highly charged electrons also can be the result of dysfunction of the immune pathway.

4. Insulin resistance, which leads to diabetes, is a mechanism involved in many chronic diseases including FMS and CFS. This is why a low-sugar diet is recommended.

All of the pathways mentioned in this chapter are involved in fatigue syndromes. As one treats the underlying illness, these pathophysiological events are resolved, thus restoring energy to the cells and reversing the fatigue. Sometimes, however, one must simply treat the pathophysiologic mechanism such as oxidative injury, the immune storm or the sludging of blood in the small capillaries, in hopes of discovering the causative agent later. In doing so, one may call it improvement but not recovery.

When it comes to chronic fatigue, many clinicians are perplexed and hard-pressed to find a diagnosis and a treatment.

Recovery involves treating the causative agent and resolving the underlying mechanism, which brings balance back to the body's immune and nervous systems.

Many physicians in America are trained in treating diseases, most of which have a definite etiology and at least a partial explanation of the mechanism or the pathophysiology in which that illness occurs. But when it comes to chronic fatigue, many clinicians are perplexed and hard-pressed to find a diagnosis and a treatment.

Simon Wessely, in an excellent paper, states that "the symptoms of fatigue remain elusive and fascinating," but he adds that the symptom itself is held in low esteem by physicians and that the presence of fatigue gives little specific diagnostic information.[4] Since virtually every medical and psychiatric disease produces fatigue, it is not viewed with great concern. Fatigue is ubiquitous and cannot be objectively measured, which frustrates the average physician. Indeed, one must do lab and X-ray tests to rule out classic diseases that produce fatigue; but when test results reveal no diagnosis, many physicians (and family members) view this with suspicion and believe the patient has an emotional problem.

I want to emphasize a statement made by Dr. Majid Ali in a 1992 address to the Academy of Otolaryngologic Allergy: "Chronic fatigue illnesses will be the scourge of the twenty-first century." Those doctors who are willing to step out of the boundaries of some traditional textbooks will be able to meet the demand of the growing number of people with this condition. There are some answers in the traditional textbooks, but these textbook answers are limited. One must go beyond textbook answers and have some knowledge of molecular biology and receptor kinetics, and one must simply be open-minded. In the history of medicine, those who thought outside the box of traditional medicine were those who made medical discoveries and were able to help their patients more proactively.

Equally important is having compassion for the patient so that along with an accurate diagnosis and treatment, you can give sympathy to the person whose life has become devastated.

Believe the patient. Treat the patient, not the lab results. Someone asked an experienced elderly country doctor what he considered to be the most important treatment for those with chronic illness. His simple answer was love, self-giving love. But then the questioner asked, "What if it doesn't work?" The physician said, "Double the dose."

Be sympathetic, love as brothers, be compassionate and humble. . . . To this you were called so that you may inherit a blessing.

1 PETER 3:8-9

CHAPTER 3

CHRONIC FATIGUE SYNDROME

In repentance and rest is your salvation, in quietness and trust is your strength.

ISAIAH 30:15

Yuppie flu, nervous exhaustion, Epstein-Barr viral syndrome, myalgic encephalomyelitis (ME)—these are some of the names that have been given to the condition commonly called chronic fatigue syndrome (CFS). Because it affects multiple systems of the body, it is labeled a syndrome, meaning a number of symptoms occurring together. It is a poorly understood illness with no proven single cause, but there are many treatment options that can significantly improve your health.

SYMPTOMS

In 1994, the Centers for Disease Control (CDC) in Atlanta recommended the following criteria for diagnosing chronic fatigue syndrome (CFS) or chronic fatigue immune deficiency syndrome (CFIDS):

- Extreme fatigue that persists for six months or more, does not resolve with bed rest and causes at least a 50 percent reduction in activity
- Exclusion of other illnesses causing similar symptoms (for instance, other medical disorders known to cause fatigue, major depressive illness, medication that causes fatigue as a side effect, and alcohol or substance abuse)

Additionally, the patient must have four of the following eight major symptoms:

- Sore throat
- Tender or swollen lymph glands
- Generalized muscle discomfort
- Migratory joint pain without swelling
- Fatigue worsened by exercise (postexertional malaise lasting over 24 hours)
- Headaches of a new type, pattern or severity
- Substantial impairment in short-term memory or concentration
- Sleep disturbance (nonrefreshing sleep)

In addition to the eight primary defining symptoms of CFS, the following are other symptoms characteristic of CFS. The frequencies of occurrence of these symptoms vary from 20 to 50 percent among CFS patients.

- Confusion, brain fog
- Dizziness, light-headedness

- Increased allergic reactions
- Food/chemical sensitivities
- Extreme sensitivities to noise, light, heat and cold
- Intestinal problems/abdominal pain
- Muscle spasms/twitches
- Achy, flulike feeling
- Muscle weakness
- Fever or chills
- Alcohol intolerance
- Bloating
- Chest pain
- Chronic cough
- Dry eyes or mouth
- Earaches
- Irregular heartbeat
- Jaw pain
- Nausea
- Night sweats
- Shortness of breath
- Skin sensations (tingling, burning)
- Psychological problems (depression, anxiety, panic)[1]

These symptoms are clinical criteria. CFS patients may have all of these symptoms or just a few. Depending on the severity of the symptoms, CFS can make it difficult for a sufferer to continue carrying on with a normal life. Physical and mental tasks may become so challenging that the ability to function diminishes dramatically. For some CFS patients, the lack of energy is so profound that getting out of bed is a major accomplishment. One patient described the

For some CFS patients, the lack of energy is so profound that getting out of bed is a major accomplishment.

extent of her debilitation in this way:

> I felt like my mind and body were on a dimmer switch. With the smallest mental or physical exertion, my energy level would fade until I couldn't function. Lifting my arms to wash my hair was a daunting task. After showering, I would need to lay down and rest. For many months, I didn't have the strength to talk on the phone. I never realized how much energy it takes to carry on a conversation! Driving was almost impossible. Not only was I too weak, but my reactions were very slow, my vision was blurry, and I couldn't remember where I was going. I tried to cook, but the mental and physical effort wore me out, and several times I left a pot on the stove, forgetting what I was doing. The inability to do much of anything was extremely depressing. I had gone from being a busy mom and wife with a demanding career and many fulfilling church activities to a seemingly invalid life. I felt like I had a terrible flu combined with jet lag and Alzheimer's, and I thought I would never get better. That was three years ago. Thankfully, today, I am much improved and able to live a fairly "normal" life, with one major difference—I no longer take for granted the ability to remain vertical for most of the day!

The wife of another CFS patient, who has since recovered and is now a managing editor for a major Christian publisher, wrote the following words in a letter to a friend who had recently been diagnosed with CFS:

> At the beginning of his illness, my husband was very discouraged. We had a wonderful doctor then, one who did not doubt the diagnosis of CFIDS at all. He was willing

to do a great deal of research for us. He tried one therapy, and when it failed, he'd try another. But before long, we realized that the standard medical community was basically unprepared to help us with this challenge.

My husband went on antidepressants, which made him much worse and caused him to gain a lot of weight. We went the herbal and homeopathic route, which helped for about three weeks before it failed. His CFIDS leaned toward the candida variety, so the anti-candida diet (no starches, yeast or sugar) did a lot of good but was nearly impossible to stay on for any length of time. Sugar, sunlight, preservatives and chemicals all worsened his condition immediately. I even had to use baking soda and vinegar as my only cleaning solutions for a time because the chemicals in my cleaners would make him worse. To this day, he will have an immediate reaction if he drinks a diet soda.

He had up and down days. It was my wish that he would rest on his up days to conserve his strength for his down days, but after a dozen down days in a row, he would want to go out and do something on an up day. Of course, then the exhaustion that set in and the worsening of his symptoms that followed depressed him. It was a very nasty cycle.

One of the hardest things for me, the spouse of a CFIDS patient, was understanding his strange memory problems. He played rotisserie baseball in those days on the computer. He could remember how many outs a certain player scored three weeks ago in a certain game, but could not remember if he had washed his hair while he was still in the shower.

My advice to you is to let the body determine the day. Use paper plates. The environment will survive. Wear your clothes until they stand up and walk themselves to the laundry. Every day do one thing that makes you feel human, but only one thing. Get help from your church or friends for the cooking and cleaning. Relax and don't worry about "feeling normal" right now. There may be no normal days for a while. The sooner you relax into that thought, the easier the down days will be. I don't have any magical combination of treatments that worked, other than "try everything and keep what works for you." And I *can* assure you that your "going-crazy" feeling is part of your illness.

I'm not going to preach at you about God trying to get your attention by making you sick. That's just stupid, and it was preached to us when my husband was sick. I'm not going to dismiss *any* symptom of yours as psychosomatic or laziness—another comment we heard a lot of in those days. When you start wondering what God's will is in all this and questioning the purpose of your existence, just think what a great minister you will be to others with CFIDS!

FACTS

Over the past decade, CFS research has shown the following:

- CFS symptoms generally have a sudden onset and are most severe for the first year.
- The clinical course of CFS varies considerably among persons who have the disorder; the actual percentage of patients who recover is unknown, and even the definition of what should be considered recovery is subject to debate. Some patients recover to the point that they can resume work and other activities but continue to

experience various or periodic CFS symptoms. Some
patients recover completely with time, and some grow
progressively worse.

- CFS often follows a cyclical course, alternating between
periods of illness and relative well-being. The course of
recovery is usually marked by periods of intermittent
relapse and improvement.

- In a recent study the CDC conducted in the Seattle
area, it was found that 59 percent of CFS patients were
female, and the average onset age of this group was 30.
The highest incidence was in women 20-50 years old,
although cases were found among all segments of the
population, including teenagers and children. More
than 80 percent had an advanced education. The incidence was 75 to 265 cases per 100,000 people. An earlier study in San Francisco found a similar level of 200
cases per 100,000.[2]

RECOGNITION

In 1984, Dr. Bill Cheney and Dr. Peterson investigated an unusual outbreak of a flulike illness in Incline Village, California.[3]
Approximately 200 people out of a population of 20,000 suc-
cumbed to what appeared to be a viral illness with symptoms of
sore throat, low-grade fever, body aches, brain fog and GI symptoms of nausea, vomiting and diarrhea. Well, that's not a big
deal in medicine, is it? After all, the flu is the most common
infection we see in medical offices across the nation. However,
this illness lasted far beyond the usual 7 to 14 days of typical
influenza. Dr. Cheney and Dr. Peterson, both immunologists,
studied the situation, looking at things such as water supply,
food intake, air quality and other epidemiological parameters.
No cause could be found. Tests (such as on stool, sputum and

blood samples) were performed on the town population but revealed nothing out of the ordinary—except the individuals had high levels of the Epstein-Barr virus. The patients were labeled as having Epstein-Barr viral syndrome, or yuppie flu. Their lifestyles were active, many had very good exercise habits, and others were leaders in their communities and churches. Depression and group hysteria were two explanations given by some psychologists, but why would 200 people simultaneously become depressed? And if it was group hysteria, the group has now expanded to over 2 million people nationwide.

As Drs. Cheney and Peterson continued their investigation into this mystery, they were asked to leave the town. Although some townspeople said the doctors were quacks, the underlying motivation for being asked to leave was probably economics. Incline Village is a tourist town and a mysterious epidemic wasn't good for business. Dr. Cheney then moved to Charlotte, North Carolina, and founded a research and treatment center for Epstein-Barr viral syndrome. I highly respect Dr. Cheney and his willingness to risk his reputation to be involved in the diagnosis and treatment of this illness.

A number of other researchers and clinicians subsequently became interested in this new syndrome, and the study and understanding of CFS began to grow. In 1988, two important facts were revealed:

1. Epstein-Barr virus levels are elevated in about half of the American population, suggesting that they meant very little in the diagnosis of this illness. Therefore, EBV *may* be one of the culprits in the cause of the syndrome, but not exclusively.
2. Another name for the illness, chronic fatigue syndrome, was proposed. Major and minor criteria were developed to diagnose the illness. Symptoms and

signs of the illness became the acceptable means for defining CFS, not lab results and X rays.[4]

The CDC in Atlanta, after previously rejecting Dr. Cheney's ideas, was now actively involved in determining clear-cut criteria for the diagnosis of the syndrome. Since then, major research has brought more understanding about CFS, including findings of related hormonal, immune and neurological mechanisms involved. The exact cause is still unknown; however, possible causes have been identified and treatments standardized.

POSSIBLE CAUSES

In my own practice, I have never seen a lazy CFS patient. Before succumbing to the illness, they are usually active (maybe too active), perhaps not getting adequate sleep and rest and, in some cases, not eating healthy foods. Many might be called workaholics.

I believe there are three main factors for developing CFS:

I have never seen a lazy CFS patient. Before succumbing to the illness, they are usually active (maybe too active), perhaps not getting adequate sleep and rest and, in some cases, not eating healthy foods.

1. Hereditary predisposition (sensitive nervous system, immune deficiencies, endocrine system abnormalities and brain chemical imbalance)

2. Cumulative chronic stress (long-term exposure to physical or mental stressors such as toxins, poor diet, lack of exercise, negative emotions, work or family pressures, sleep deprivation, and so on)

3. Acute debilitating event (serious injury, surgery, emotional crisis, severe flu or other transient traumatic
condition)

Generally, the onset of chronic fatigue is definite and many
times occurs after some form of infectious illness. (This is not to
say that CFS is *caused* by the illness; a virus may just be the straw
that broke the camel's back.) If your symptoms began with a
severe virus, your doctor probably treated you with antibiotics,
which did not improve your symptoms. When talking to your
doctor, you might have had difficulty describing the nature of
your fatigue. It is something most of us have not experienced, even
with serious illness. It is truly a liquid, heavy exhaustion. The unrelenting fatigue caused a disruption of your activities. After a period of time, you may have tried to exercise, but the exertion made
you feel worse. You likely experienced insomnia and a lack of restful sleep, which is very debilitating and causes many patients to
rely on over-the-counter sleep aids or prescriptions. But the
fatigue still persisted. After several months, perhaps you began to
seek other medical help and received no specific diagnosis.

Many times, CFS patients are offered antidepressants or are
sent to a psychiatrist. If you were diagnosed with major depression, let me emphasize that CFS is not caused by depression.
However, one may experience secondary depression due to
fatigue and other debilitating symptoms. The demonstrable differences between depression and CFS are as follows:

- Pituitary-adrenal axis is down-regulated in CFS and
up-regulated in depression.[5]
- There is more personality change in depression than
CFS.[6]
- Overall differences in immune parameters between CFS
and depression clearly exist.[7]

• Depression is usually helped by exercise, while CFS is worsened by strenuous activity.

The proven cause or causes of CFS remain unknown, despite a vigorous search. While a single cause for CFS may yet be identified, another possibility is that CFS represents a common endpoint of disease resulting from multiple precipitating causes. Therefore, any of the possible causes listed below, or a combination of them, may be the root of your problem. These largely unrelated possible causes are not mutually exclusive.

Infectious Agents

Due in part to its similarity to chronic mononucleosis, CFS was initially thought to be caused by a viral infection, most probably the Epstein-Barr virus. It now seems clear that CFS cannot be caused exclusively by EBV or by any other single recognized infectious disease agent. No firm association between infection with any known human pathogen and CFS has been established. However, the possibility remains that CFS may have multiple causes, in which case some viruses or other infectious agents might have a contributory role for a subset of CFS cases.

The virus most closely associated with CFS is HHV-6 (a herpes virus). When treated appropriately for this virus, many infected patients go into remission.[8] Lyme disease, a spirochete bacteria, is also a major cause of CFS and FMS.

The first indication of CFS may be when the patient succumbs to an acute illness— usually viral.

Immune System

As stated previously, the first indication of CFS may be when the patient succumbs to an acute illness—usually viral. When the fatigue and flulike symptoms persist, the implication is that a dysfunction of the immune system is involved.

As mentioned in chapter 2, the immune system has two primary functions. One is repair—the ability to fix what is broken, such as a fractured bone or a cut on the skin. The second major function is protection. The immune system protects our bodies by attacking and killing outside invaders such as viruses, bacteria and fungi. It also attacks internal invaders such as cancer cells. Immune dysfunction (or autoimmune disease) occurs when the body's killer cells overreact and begin to attack healthy cells. Some investigators have observed antiself antibodies in many CFS patients, which is a hallmark of autoimmune disease. However, no associated tissue damage typical of autoimmune disease has been described in patients with CFS. Additionally, the opportunistic infections or increased risk for cancer observed in persons with immunodeficiency diseases is not observed in CFS patients.

One intriguing hypothesis is that various triggering events such as stress or a viral infection may lead to the chronic overproduction of cytokines and then to CFS. Cytokines ("cell-movers") are the messengers of the immune system. They are the communication system that keeps all the elements of the immune system working together effectively. Cytokines are the signaling chemicals that regulate cell growth, immunity, inflammation and tissue repair. Because of their role in causing inflammation, they are called proinflammatory. Inflammation in a healthy person is a natural response to injury or infection and is part of the healing process. However, when under any type of prolonged stress, the body continues to produce cytokines and the process of inflammation does not shut down properly. Research has shown that elevated cytokine levels can also be caused by hormone imbalances and sleep deprivation.

Most CFS patients show evidence of unusual immune activation, as demonstrated by an increased number of activated cytoxic T cells, as well as elevated levels of circulating cytokines. Many researchers believe that an altered immune system functioning along with chronic inflammation can either be the cause of or contribute to CFS.[9] Besides inflammation, an excess of cytokines can cause flulike symptoms including fever, achiness and fatigue—typical symptoms of CFS.

Finally, several studies have shown that CFS patients are more likely to have a history of allergies than are healthy controls. Allergy could be one predisposing factor for CFS, but it cannot be the only one, since not all CFS patients have it.

Hypothalamic-Pituitary-Adrenal (HPA) Axis

Multiple laboratory studies have suggested that the central nervous system may have an important role in CFS. Physical or emotional stress, which is commonly reported as a pre-onset condition in CFS patients, activates the hypothalamic-pituitary-adrenal axis, or HPA axis, leading to an increased release of cortisol and other hormones. Cortisol and corticotrophin-releasing hormones (CRH), which also are produced during the activation of the HPA axis, influence the immune system and many other body systems. They also may affect several aspects of behavior. Recent studies revealed that CFS patients often produce lower levels of cortisol than do healthy controls. This may be termed adrenal exhaustion. (Before the onset of the illness, constant stress likely causes elevated levels of cortisol. At some point, the adrenals became overwhelmed and production of cortisol drops.) Cortisol suppresses inflammation and cellular immune activation, and reduced levels might relax constraints on inflammatory processes and immune cell activation. Because the altered cortisol levels noted in CFS cases usually fall within the accepted range of normal, they cannot be used as a diagnostic marker for an individual with CFS. Recent studies have concluded that low levels of cortisol itself are not directly responsible for symptoms of CFS and that hormonal replacement (with hydro-cortisone) is not an effective treatment. However, important research continues in this largely unexplored field.

Neurally Mediated Hypotension

Neurally mediated hypotension (NMH) is a condition in which the body has difficulty regulating blood pressure, especially when standing upright. The autonomic nervous system, which controls heart rate and blood pressure, misinterprets what the body needs during periods of upright posture and sends a message to the heart to lower blood pressure. Normally, the heart would speed up and the blood vessels in the legs would tighten, leading to an increase in blood pressure. However, in many CFS patients, when the blood pressure first begins to fall after standing for a few minutes, the heart slows down and the blood vessels in the legs loosen. The blood flow to the brain is then reduced. This drop in blood pressure can lead to weakness, dizziness, sweating, vision disturbance, difficulty with concentration and a feeling of faintness. NMH typically occurs after exercise, periods of standing or exposure to heat. Many CFS patients therefore experience lightheadedness or worsened fatigue when they stand in a warm environment such as in a hot shower.[10]

Some researchers claim that CFS is caused by NMH. However, many physicians who specialize in treating CFS believe that faulty blood pressure regulation is a sign of adrenal malfunction—simply another symptom of CFS and not its cause. NMH cannot be diagnosed with typical blood pressure readings. It requires a tilt-table test that continually monitors blood pressure for 45 minutes while the patient is slowly tilted from a horizontal to a nearly vertical position. One study observed that 96 percent of adults with a clinical diagnosis of CFS developed hypotension during tilt-table testing, compared to 29 percent of healthy controls. Tilt-table testing also provoked characteristic

CFS symptoms in the patients. If test results are positive (a significant drop in blood pressure and pulse rate), treatment may consist of medications to boost blood pressure and prevent the heartbeat from slowing down. A placebo-controlled trial of NMH medications for CFS patients is now in progress. Increasing intake of water and salt can also improve the symptoms of NMH. Because water and salt contribute to a higher blood volume, they help to keep the pressure elevated. However, before increasing salt intake, CFS patients should consult with a physician, because high-salt diets may endanger some individuals.

Neurochemistry Imbalance

The brain and nervous system also play a central role in fatigue.[11] The brain itself can become inflamed, as was described in a classic paper in the CFIDS Journal of 1992. This theory is basically unchanged today and has general scientific acceptance.

It may be surprising to some that the brain can actually injure itself. Just as the immune system attacks itself when proinflammatory cytokines are up- regulated and overreact, injury to nerve cells can result when certain chemicals in the brain are out of balance.

GABA, serotonin and magnesium are the calming chemicals in the brain and nervous system, while norepinephrine, dopamine, glutamate and NMDA are the excitatory chemicals. The chemicals that are important in CFS, and also in opposition to one another, are GABA and NMDA. If GABA prevails over the NMDA receptors, a progression from sedation to sleep to coma can occur. If NMDA prevails, a progression from mania to seizures can occur.[12] If the firing rate of the NMDA neurons overwhelms GABA firing (as may be the case in CFS), the brain is in such a hyperexcitable state that toxicity occurs—the brain harms itself. This overstimulation of brain activity prevents the patient from obtaining adequate sleep and rest—one of the major problems with CFS. This brain hyperactivity may be compared to an automobile that is racing 100 mph and is unable to slow down. This causes unusual, accelerated wear and tear on the engine, the tires and the body of the car. The brain is much the same. It is in a state of such hypervigilance that fatigue results—a type of fatigue that actually inhibits sleep instead of promoting it. Your body is extremely tired, but your brain chemicals are not allowing it truly to rest. However, when there is an increase in GABA and/or a decrease in NMDA excitability, balance is restored and symptoms improve.

Nutritional Deficiency

There is no published scientific evidence that CFS is caused by a nutritional deficiency. Many patients do report intolerance for certain substances that may be found in foods or over-the-counter medications, such as alcohol or the artificial sweetener aspartame. While evidence is currently lacking for nutritional defects in CFS patients, it also should be added that a balanced diet can be conducive to better health in general and would be expected to have beneficial effects in any chronic illness.

TREATMENTS

A variety of therapeutic approaches have been described as benefiting patients with chronic fatigue syndrome. Since no cause for CFS has been identified and the pathophysiology remains unknown, treatment programs are directed at relief of symptoms, the goal being for the patient to regain some level of pre-existing function and well-being. Although desirable, a rapid return to pre-illness health may not be realistic, and patients who expect this prompt recovery and do not experience it may exacerbate their symptoms because of overexertion and frustration, and may worsen instead of improving.

Decisions regarding treatment for CFS or any chronically fatiguing illness should be made only in consultation with a health-care provider. The physician, together with the patient, can develop an individually tailored program that provides the greatest benefit. This treatment program should be based on an assessment of the patient's overall medical condition and current symptoms and should be modified over time on the basis of regular follow-up and assessment of the patient's changing condition. Currently, most health-care providers with experience in treating persons with CFS use some combination of the therapies discussed below.

Some proposed treatments are unproven and may be harmful. Therapy should not aggravate existing symptoms or create new ones. It should not mask another illness that needs identification and specific treatment. Additionally, therapy should not impose an excessive financial burden on the patient.

I have been able to help most CFS patients using both traditional and novel strategies learned over the years. There are physicians throughout the United States who also understand CFS and have very good treatment responses. *There is hope!*

Pharmacologic Therapy

Pharmacologic therapy is directed toward the relief of specific symptoms experienced by the individual patient. Patients with CFS appear particularly sensitive to many medications, especially those that affect the central nervous system, and they often have exaggerated or opposite reactions to drugs. Thus, the usual treatment strategy is to begin with a very low dose and to increase the dosage gradually as necessary and as tolerated. It is important to remember that the use of any drug for symptom relief should be attempted only if an underlying cause for the symptom in question has not been found. The best example is the use of a sleep-enhancing medication for nonrestorative sleep. Although you may feel that you sleep better, the cause of the sleep disorder remains obscured and is not being treated. It also is important to remember that all medications can cause side effects, which may lead to new symptoms.

Prescription Medications

Nonsteroidal Anti-Inflammatory Drugs. These drugs are used to relieve pain in some CFS patients. Some are available as over-the-counter medications. Examples include naproxen (Aleve, Anaprox, Naprosen), ibuprofen (Advil, Bayer Select, Motrin, Nuprin) and piroxicam (Feldene). Prescription drugs include celecoxib (Celebrex) and refecoxib (Vioxx). These medications are generally safe when used as directed but can cause a variety of adverse effects including kidney damage, gastrointestinal bleeding, abdominal pain, nausea and vomiting. Some patients may become dependent on some of these agents. In general, the medications listed above are of little value in treating CFS. I have found them to be more effective in treating arthritis or general body aches and pains.

Low-Dose Tricyclic Antidepressants. Tricyclic agents (TCAs) may be prescribed for CFS patients to improve sleep and to relieve mild, generalized pain. Examples include doxepin (Adapin, Sinequan), amitriptyline (Elavil), imipramine (Tofranil), trazodone (Desyrel) and nortriptyline (Pamelor). Effective dosages are often much lower than those used to treat depression. Some adverse reactions include dry mouth, drowsiness, weight gain and elevated heart rate.

Other Antidepressants. Examples of antidepressants used to treat patients with CFS include selective serotonin reuptake inhibitors (SSRIs) such as fluoxetine (Prozac), sertraline (Zoloft), paroxetine (Paxil), citalapian (Celexa), venlafaxine (Effexor) and bupropion (Wellbutrin). These may be effective in correcting the various brain-chemical imbalances that are a problem for many CFS patients. Wellbutrin has been the most effective for many of my patients because it increases dopamine and norepinephrine, two brain chemicals that are low in CFS. However, each patient is unique and no one medication or dosage is right for everyone. A number of adverse reactions—varying with the specific drug—may be experienced, including agitation, sleep disturbances and, in rare cases, increased fatigue. There also is a documented discontinuation syndrome associated with some antidepressants, especially Effexor and Paxil. To lessen the unpleasant effects of discontinuation, work closely with your physician to taper your dosage slowly.

Anxiolytic Agents. Anxiolytic agents may be used to treat symptoms of anxiety in CFS patients. Examples include alprazolam (Xanax) and lorazepam (Ativan). Clonazepam (Klonopin) is another member of this family of drugs that is used to control exaggerated nervous-system problems such as vertigo, a burning sensation, exaggerated tenderness of the skin and restless limb movements. These drugs all down-regulate the NMDA brain receptor sites and conversely up-regulate the GABA receptors. As one increases the dosage of these drugs past the balance point, then sedation and sleep usually will occur. If a normal person is drowsy or fatigued and takes Klonopin or Xanax, he or she falls asleep. However, when a CFS patient takes the same medication, there is a paradoxical lessening of fatigue and brain fog and an increase in cognition. Therefore, I believe it is the NMDA/GABA theory that explains the major pathophysiologic mechanisms in CFS. However, anxiolytic agents should not be used in the general treatment of CFS, because they are habit forming. Other brain chemical-balancing drugs such as antidepressants are more suited for long-term use in CFS. Common adverse reactions include sedation, amnesia and symptoms accompanying acute withdrawal (i.e., insomnia, abdominal and muscle cramps, vomiting, sweating, tremors and convulsions).

Antimicrobials. An infectious cause for CFS has not been identified, and antibiotics, antivirals and antifungal agents should not be prescribed for treatment of CFS unless the patient has been diagnosed with a concurrent infection. A controlled trial of the antiviral drug acyclovir found no benefit in the treatment of CFS patients, but transfer factor (described later in this chapter) has been found very useful. Indiscriminant use of antimicrobials can have myriad adverse effects including increasing the risk for resistant organisms.

Anti-Allergy Therapy. Some CFS patients have histories of allergy, and these symptoms may flare up periodically. Nonsedating antihistamines may be helpful for CFS patients with allergies. Examples include desloratadine (Clarinex), fexofenadine (Allegra) and ceterizine (Zyrtec). Sedating antihistamines such as Benadryl can also be of benefit to patients at bedtime. The tricyclic antidepressants already mentioned also have potent antihistamine effects. Allergy shots along with another allergy technique described later—in the "To the Physician" section—have been my most effective treatments. I have been amazed at the positive results.

Blood Pressure Therapy. CFS does not respond to treatment with antihypotensive or antitachycardic drugs, and general use of such medications may be harmful. However, such medications may be useful in specific circumstances. For example, fludrocortisone (Florinef) has been prescribed for CFS patients who have had a positive tilt-table test, although controlled studies have not found Florinef alone effective in the general treatment of CFS patients. Beta-blockers such as atenolol (Tenormin) have also been prescribed for patients with neurally mediated hypotension. Midodrine (Proamatine), an agent that directly increases blood pressure, may be useful in selected patients identified by an abnormal tilt-table test. Increased salt and water intake also is recommended for these patients but should be done only under supervision of a health-care provider. Adverse reactions include elevated blood pressure and fluid retention. Some cardiologists recommend antidepressants such as Celexa or Lexipro, but I have found Effexor or Wellbutrin to work best, since their side effects include elevated blood pressure.

Experimental Drugs and Treatments

Dehydroepiandrosterone (DHEA) was reported in preliminary studies to improve symptoms in some patients. However, in subsequent studies, this finding was not confirmed, so the use of DHEA in patients should be regarded as experimental. DHEA up-regulates GABA, an important brain chemical in this syndrome. Its use should be limited to patients with documented abnormalities in DHEA levels and function. The use of natural progesterone has proven to be beneficial in some women with CFS. Both DHEA and progesterone have positive effects on dopamine levels in the brain. They can be obtained in cream form from compounding pharmacists.

Nonpharmacologic Therapy

Physical Activity. An appropriate amount of physical activity is required by everyone for physical and emotional well-being. Patients with CFS are no exception. Sufficient rest is crucial to recovery from CFS. However, inactivity can lead to physical deconditioning, which may cause a downward spiral of muscle weakness, cardiovascular function and depression. To avoid deconditioning, modest regular exercise such as walking is essential. Even on days you are feeling too exhausted to take a short walk, try to move a little. Fold a load of laundry, bring in a log for the fire, or brush the dog. A prolonged lack of movement can make your fatigue worse, but so can overexertion. Therefore, a key consideration for patients with CFS is to know how much to do and when to stop the activity. Regardless of the level of activity a patient with CFS may attempt, the most important guideline is to avoid increasing the level of fatigue.

Pace yourself carefully and avoid unusual physical or emotional stress. Any activity can be counterproductive if it increases fatigue or pain. A regular, manageable daily routine helps avoid the push-crash phenomenon characterized by overexertion during periods of better health, followed by a relapse of symptoms perhaps initiated by the excessive activity.

Although patients should be as active as possible, physicians may need to explain the disorder to employers and family members, advising them to make allowances as needed.

Other helpful physical therapies include massage, nonforce chiropractic and therapeutic touch. These passive therapies may contribute to feeling better, but they are most effective when combined with patient-generated activity, including aquatic therapy, light exercise (adapted to personal capabilities) and gentle stretching.

Education. Learning about what CFS is and what it is not is a critical component of therapy. This approach includes learning how to adjust activities and behaviors that may aggravate the illness. A formal method to impart this information is known as cognitive behavioral therapy.

Cognitive behavioral therapy has been shown to facilitate patient coping and to allow increased activities without triggering increased symptoms. Regular sessions with a qualified psychologist who is familiar with CFS can be very beneficial.

Any chronic illness, including CFS, can affect the patient's family. Family education may foster good communication and reduce the adverse effect of CFS on the family. The Internet is a helpful resource for finding current information about CFS. However, any website with the primary purpose of selling you a product may not contain the most reliable content. Look for sites that are sponsored by university medical centers, professional medical organizations and government agencies such as the CDC (these sites usually have a ".gov" or ".org" suffix).

Nutritional Therapy. Many CFS patients have multiple food sensitivities, which many experts believe are not the same as true allergies. However, the subject is controversial among allergists, some of whom assert that the sensitivities are true allergies. Sensitivities can be temporary, caused by an overactive immune system that reacts to certain nonharmful chemicals and nutrients as if they were toxins. The foods most likely to cause problems include the following:

- Wheat
- Yeast
- Milk
- Sugar
- Peanuts
- Corn
- Eggs
- Citrus fruits
- Soy products
- Caffeine
- Alcohol
- Food additives (preservatives and flavorings)

Any type of food intolerance may cause digestive system problems including bloating, belching, diarrhea and gas. Certain foods and additives also can cause histamine reactions such as headache, runny nose, hives and itching. If you experience any of these symptoms, a systematic elimination program can be helpful to find the foods that are the offenders. For at least a week, eliminate one food item at a time from your diet and note whether the symptoms disappear. Then reintroduce the food item and see if the symptoms return. A total exclusion of wheat and dairy products helps many patients as they recover. Alcohol and caffeine must be avoided because of their effect on the nervous system.

Sugar is problematic for CFS patients because of its up-and-down effect on the body. A CFS patient may have normal glucose tolerance test results, meaning blood-sugar levels are not unusually low; however, the patient *feels* every change in the level of blood sugar more than the average person. Blood-sugar fluctuations can cause decreased energy levels, dizziness, headache, agitation, shakiness and mood swings. Therefore, the CFS patient should attempt to keep the blood-sugar level as even as possible.

Sugar is problematic for CFS patients because of its up-and-down effect on the body.

This is accomplished by eating frequent small meals and avoiding sugar and simple carbohydrates (most white foods, including white bread, white rice and potatoes, which turn to sugar very quickly in your body). One reason for CFS patients' intolerance of sugars is the common coexistence of yeast or bacterial overgrowth in their intestines (see chapter 6).

Complex carbohydrates (vegetables and whole grains) should be consumed with some sort of protein and small amounts of fat, which help to metabolize the carbohydrates at a slow, steady rate. Foods that usually are well tolerated and nutritious are poultry, fish, most fruits, vegetables, brown rice and plain yogurt with active cultures. Even those with sensitivities to dairy products can usually tolerate yogurt.

Eating foods high in antioxidants (vitamins A, C and E) will help prevent cell damage caused by free radicals. Remember the example of lemon juice preventing a cut apple from turning brown. Many common foods—especially colorful fruits and vegetables—have this type of antioxidant property. Here is a list of foods high in antioxidants:

- Carrots
- Dark-green leafy vegetables
- Sweet potatoes
- Apricots
- Red peppers
- Citrus fruits
- Purple fruits
- Tomatoes
- Broccoli
- Nuts
- Whole grains
- Vegetable oils
- Others: garlic, turmeric, green tea and soy

The following foods are particularly beneficial for countering cytokine-caused inflammation and the accompanying CFS symptoms. They help maintain proper cytokine balance.

- Coldwater fish (i.e., salmon, trout, swordfish, cod and halibut)
- Fresh pineapple and papaya
- Spinach
- Blueberries
- Strawberries
- Onions

Dietary Supplements and Herbal Preparations. A variety of dietary supplements and herbal preparations are claimed to have potential benefits for CFS patients. With few exceptions, the effectiveness of these remedies for treating CFS has not been evaluated in controlled trials. Contrary to common belief, the "natural" origin of a product does not ensure safety. Dietary supplements and herbal preparations can have potentially serious side effects, and some can interfere or interact with prescription medications. CFS patients should seek the advice of their health-care provider before using any nonprescribed remedy.

Preparations that have been claimed to have benefit for CFS patients include adenosine monophosphate, coenzyme Q-10, germanium, glutathione, iron, magnesium sulfate, melatonin, NADH, selenium, l-tryptophan, zinc and vitamins B12, C, E and A. An early CFS study found reduced red blood cell magnesium sulfate in CFS patients, but two subsequent studies have found no difference between patients and healthy controls. The therapeutic value of all these preparations for CFS has not been validated.

Plants are known sources of many pharmacological materials. However, unrefined herbal preparations contain variable levels of the active compound and may contain many irrelevant, potentially harmful substances. Preparations that have been claimed to benefit CFS patients include astralagus, borage seed oil, bromelain, comfrey, echinacea, garlic, ginkgo biloba, ginseng, primrose oil, quercetin, St. John's wort and shiitake mushroom extract. Only primrose oil was evaluated in a controlled study, and the beneficial effects noted in CFS patients have not been independently confirmed. Some herbal preparations, notably comfrey and high-dose ginseng, have recognized harmful effects.

Many of my patients have responded well to these supplements: B12 shots, magnesium, zinc, coenzyme Q-10, melatonin (at night) and omega-3 EFAs. Magnesium and melatonin are taken at bedtime in three to six milligram doses. I believe omega-3 (fish oil) EFAs should be taken by every CFS patient. The EFAs are vital for healthy cell membranes—especially in the central nervous system—and are essential for immune system balance. Antioxidant vitamins (A, C and E) are important for preventing cell damage caused by free radicals.

Rest. A century ago, people suffering from nervous exhaustion were prescribed a rest cure, which meant retreating to some nonstressful location for a long period of time. Sound good? To a large degree, recovery from CFS requires rest—mental and physical. Most patients have times when they can't get out of bed, so rest is not a choice. But lying in bed is not the only form of rest needed. While resting your body, your mind can still be in turmoil. If you are worrying about your health and obsessing about every new symptom, true rest is not occurring. Finding ways to rest and slow down your mind is vital. In the psalms, we hear David cry out to God about his pain and anguish and exhaustion. The source of David's replenished strength and healing is always the same: "My soul finds rest in God alone" (Ps. 62:1). Jesus speaks to the hearts of everyone who is worn out when He says:

While resting your body, your mind can still be in turmoil. Finding ways to rest and slow down your mind is vital.

> Come to me, all you who are weary and burdened, and I will give you rest. Take my yoke upon you and learn from me, for I am gentle and humble in heart, and you will find rest for your souls (Matt. 11: 28-29).

Optimal physical rest is something that all patients need to gauge for themselves. When you feel so exhausted that you can barely walk, sitting and reading or listening to the radio all day can be therapeutic. On days when you have a little more energy, do some small tasks, but sit down and rest often. Don't feel guilty because it takes you forever to unload the dishwasher. It's *okay* to set a slow pace for yourself.

When your body is tired, exercise your mind. When your mind is tired, exercise your body. But *never* attempt strenuous exercise, because it will almost always worsen your symptoms. Additionally, keep in mind that low blood sugar can make you feel so weak that you can't think or lift a finger. A nutritious snack will sometimes be more helpful than a nap.

Don't let your need for rest keep you isolated. Socializing takes a lot of energy, but it's important for your mental state. One patient said, "A night out with friends for dinner equals three days in bed." That's a choice you might have to make. If resting is always your first priority, you may become depressed from a lack of human interaction. If your priority is socializing, you may have a longer recovery. Finding a balance that doesn't worsen your condition is the key.

You may want to find a retreat center near you where you can completely rest for a week or more. Many Christian organizations provide retreats that include meals with no organized agenda other than to spend time alone with God. Catholic retreat centers especially are well known for their beautiful locations and opportunities for silent meditation.

Spiritual Healing. Illness can bring us to God in many ways. When you're lying in bed and feeling completely miserable and helpless, God can seem a million miles away, or He can be your sole comfort and hope. Talking to Him in prayer during your darkest times can foster peace of mind and bring the rest that will help strengthen and heal your body. Use those times to tell God all of your feelings, and listen quietly to His "still small voice" (1 Kings 19:12, *KJV*).

Well-meaning friends may pray for your healing and then get discouraged and wonder what's wrong if you're not better in a few weeks. Don't allow people to make you feel worse because you're not meeting their expectations of God's timetable. His healing comes in unique ways and at different times for each of us.

Reading God's promises in the Bible is a powerful reminder of His presence and care for you. You may find keeping a journal helps you to express your thoughts and record your prayers and favorite verses. The quiet, down time of illness also can provide an opportunity for introspection that has previously taken a backseat amidst your busy schedule. It's a good time to reflect on the areas of your life that might need some changes. What is really important to you? Have you been focusing on those things or letting daily problems and noncrucial issues become your priority? Have you been constantly rushing, feeling as though there's not enough time to fulfill all your obligations? Do you have relationships that have become strained? Have you asked God to help you forgive people with whom you've had conflicts? Is there an area of your life that has been causing excess stress and needs to be resolved? Even though you may not have the energy to confront problems and make major changes in your life, this can be a good time to clean house mentally. Your body has forced you to slow down. Listen to what it is trying to tell you. As mentioned more thoroughly in chapters 4 and 7, a self-imposed anxious desire to control is common in many of my CFS patients. Simply to let go and let God be in control may not be simple, but it is vital. "Be still, and know that I am God" (Ps. 46:10).

Ask God for His wisdom and help to redeem this time of suffering with a purpose only He can provide. In Joel 2:25, God says, "I will repay you for the years the locusts have eaten." What a promise! Not only is God with us during every minute of our pain and illness, but also He will not let the terrible months and years that were "eaten by locusts" go to waste.

In the following Bible passage, God is speaking to the Israelites, who were being held captive in Babylon in the year 597 B.C. In many ways, your illness may be holding you captive, and His promise is for you, too:

"For I know the plans I have for you," declares the LORD,
"plans to prosper you and not to harm you, plans to give

you hope and a future. Then you will call upon me and come and pray to me, and I will listen to you. You will seek me and find me when you seek me with all your heart. I will be found by you," declares the LORD, "and will bring you back from captivity" (Jer. 29:11-14).

CONCLUSION

Every patient is different. The human body is amazingly complicated and "wonderfully made" (Ps. 139:14). The reasons for your illness, and your reactions to various treatments, will not be exactly like other CFS patients. Therefore, you will need to work closely with your physician to discover what is most effective for you. It can be a long, frustrating process, but there's light at the end of the tunnel! A patient who has experienced almost full recovery wrote the following letter to several doctors in her community. You may relate to her experience and want to discuss with your own physician some of the following 10 issues she brings to light. Clear and honest communication will help speed up your recovery.

> I'm hoping that this letter might be helpful to those of you who treat people suffering from fibromyalgia/CFS. You see, I am one of those "difficult patients." Since no one seems to have a complete understanding of what this illness actually is or how to "cure" it, CFS can be frustrating for the doctor and the patient. Thanks for caring for us and not giving up, even though we are challenging.

> 1. **We are scared and confused.** We live each day in a frightening world of not knowing what is going on

with our bodies. It is like waking up in the middle of a live mine field every morning, wondering what body part is going to go wacko today, and what we did to trigger it. Are my head and arm jerking uncontrollably because I'm tapering off Effexor? Is my skin burning and my throat closing up because I ate some MSG? Do I have weakness and vertigo, am I bumping into walls, and are my knees buckling because of a side effect of the Wellbutrin I just started taking? Or because I overdid it yesterday by taking two walks? Sounds paranoid, I know. Feeling like you might be ambushed by your own body at any moment of the day can do that to you. Three years ago when I had my major CFS "crash" and had to stop working full time, I told my husband it felt like my brain broke (just an analogy—I know that doesn't really happen), like the master control went on red alert. Then the dominoes started falling—one previously normal body function after another—until my entire body was operating at 20 percent.

2. **We are desperate for information.** The Internet is our best friend and worst enemy. We want to understand our condition. Please give us copies of helpful articles and try to answer our questions thoroughly, so we can rely on you and not the Internet for our information. There are some good websites, but a lot of them use fear and pseudomedical jargon to get us to buy their book or remedy. Please steer your patients toward professional, reliable sites.

3. **We feel crazy, but we need to be reassured that we really aren't (permanently, anyway).** Encourage patients to find a good psychologist—not because technically we are mentally ill, but because it is very

beneficial to have help coping with a loss of health and drastic change in lifestyle. We may feel like mental cases—and you might think we are, too—but please tell us that is a normal part of CFS. And don't write us off as hypochondriacs. This illness makes it very hard not to be one. We need help learning not to obsess about all our ailments. A major component of CFS *is* its effect on one's mind (it is really, really depressing).

4. **Telling us we are not going to die of CFS is comforting, but . . .** This sounds dramatic, but on our worst days we would prefer death to a life of CFS. Please tell us we will not only *not* die, but we will most likely get better. Hope is very therapeutic. We would love to have you diagnose us with an infection or even something much worse, as strange as that seems. Anything that can be diagnosed and treated is preferable to a debilitating mystery condition that takes away your life. That's why we go chasing after cures, searching for an effective treatment.

5. **We are overly sensitive (understatement)!** I feel as though my body has lost the ability to adapt—to anything! Cold/heat, sleep/wake, changes in blood sugar, meds, changes in blood pressure (postural), hormonal changes, wind, altitude and so on—to a healthy person these are no big deal; but our bodies seem to be unusually sensitive and overreact to any change. I learned the hard way that I can only handle the very smallest doses of any medication. So start with really tiny dosages, even if it seems ridiculous. And help us not to be discouraged when we have odd or opposite reactions. We really aren't trying to be difficult. We just have unique (I sometimes think "mutant") systems. Please understand why we may seem hesitant to

try new meds. After so many terrible reactions, we're just being realistic. We also would appreciate being educated about our meds. Sometimes our minds are too befuddled to ask intelligent questions.

6. **Take a look at family patterns of sensitivities.** Some of our condition may be genetic. I was surprised to find out that back in the 1980s my older sister had many of my symptoms and was labeled hypoglycemic. I've discovered through much experimentation that lots of my symptoms are also food-triggered (MSG, alcohol, caffeine and sugar are the worst). I also found out that family members have mitral valve prolapse and autonomic nervous system overactivity, as I do. It's helped me to look at the big picture of what runs in my family and what has helped them.

7. **Be specific about the benefits of exercise.** Emphasize the downward spiral of inactivity. We are exhausted, and we hurt; and it is very hard to get going, especially when we've been told that resting will make us better. I heard Michael J. Fox say that for him, walking across a room took 10 times more energy than for the average person. Going for a walk can wipe me out for a whole day, which makes me hesitant to take a walk! But if I never move, the deconditioning that results will only make me worse. Moderation has been the key for me. If I pay attention, my body will tell me when I'm overdoing it. Warm-water exercise classes are great. They really help with the muscle aches. Gentle stretching is good. Patients can use videotapes at home to guide their stretching and breathing exercises. But just basic walking—as much as my body can handle without feeling lightheaded or shaky—has helped me the most.

8. **Stress is our number one enemy.** Help us learn how to minimize stress in our lives, because *any* stress makes us worse. One concept that really helped me is this: There is a stress/energy drain hierarchy in CFS. The most damaging is emotional stress (i.e., fear, anger, sadness, conflict and so on), then mental stress (i.e., complex thinking, conversing, trying to follow complicated directions and so on) and then physical stress (i.e., any bodily activity). If there is a choice, choose lower on the scale! Keep to a minimum any activities that cause multiple stresses. For example, going to a wedding or even a dinner party can be emotionally, mentally (talking to people) and physically (standing for a long time) stressful. Resting up for a few days ahead of time is a good idea. Or if it is too much of a drain, don't go. We need to learn how to take care of our newly limited selves. Ask questions to help us determine the stresses in our lives and how they impact our health.

9. **Encourage a creative outlet.** We can get stuck in a negative "poor me, I can't do anything" place, and low-energy creative projects can be a healthy antidote. Gardening, painting, sculpting, singing, playing an instrument, writing and quilting—whatever the person enjoys—are good outlets. Sometimes we have to force ourselves to do it, but it really does help.

10. **Nonforce chiropractic and physical therapy can be helpful.** The hard-core manipulation stuff was too much for me and made me worse, but nonforce adjustments have been beneficial. The same goes for massage. The deep-tissue kind really hurt me, but the more gentle methods are okay.

In summary, we appreciate all you try to do for us. You may not realize what an important factor you are in our recovery.[12]

TO THE PHYSICIAN

CHRONIC FATIGUE SYNDROME

Epidemiology Increasingly common

Key symptoms and history
1. Sometimes abrupt onset after viral illness or injury
2. Chronic fatigue
3. Initial sore throat and fever
4. Brain fog
5. Allergies very common

Diagnosis Challenging, must rule out other fatigue-causing illnesses

Treatment approach
1. Can be complicated
2. Unusual reactions to drugs,
3. Effective treatment varies with individuals

Prognosis
1. Poor if not diagnosed or treated wisely

Continued on next page

Continued from previous page

2. Improvement of remission probable with proper treatment
3. Spontaneous remission possible for some
4. Cycles of improvement and relapse common
5. May develop into fibromyalgia for some

To make a CFS diagnosis, the physician must first exclude, among other diseases:

- Active medical conditions such as low thyroid, and sleep problems such as narcolepsy
- Medical conditions not fully resolved (i.e., malignancies, hepatitis, Lyme disease, lupus and so on)
- Major depression and anorexia or bulimia
- Alcohol or substance abuse occurring up to two years prior to CFS and anytime afterward (CFS is excluded according to the case definition of the CDC)

Many symptoms overlap CFS, the yeast syndrome and low thyroid illness. It is incumbent upon the physician to rule out candida and hypothyroidism. If you treat either of these conditions and the patient improves, by definition they do not have CFS; they have fatigue due to that illness. Let me hasten to say that I have seen a number of people who have CFS and the yeast connection or hypothyroidism, or all three, and treating each is essential to improvement.

FMS/CHRONIC FATIGUE LAB WORKUP

First Tier

CBC, complete chemistries (CMP), ESR, ANA, U/A, Chest X ray or TB test if indicated.

Oral swab for wet prep or KOH if indicated.

Second Tier

HHV-6 titers, chlamydia or mycoplasma antibodies, provocative screen for heavy metals, immuno-toxicity screen, culture/sensitivity of nares, comprehensive stool analysis, fungal titers if indicated, allergy testing, T & B lymphocyte subsets, vaccine neutralization.

Other tests to rule out other diseases may include CT scan of chest and abdomen, MRI or spect-scan of brain.

Third Tier

Rheumatoid factors, Lyme titers (igenex labs), western blot and/or PCR, immunoglobulin levels, serum cortisol, fact test (visual contrast sensitivity test if indicated), HIV, RPR, sinus X ray, free testosterone, possibly HAM-D or other questionnaire if depression is a question (usually this is apparent and Wellbutrin and Effexor may have already been started).

TREATMENT

The treatment for chronic fatigue syndrome in our clinic is generally focused on the immunologic imbalance as well as on brain chemistry abnormalities. It is my strong belief that hyperactive central nervous and immune systems and occult adrenal exhaustion are to blame (though there is evidence of immune depression in some patients). When one understands the role of immune overactivity, NMDA receptor neurotoxicity and endocrine malfunction, a treatment plan can be devised. Remember, the hyperreactive, overwhelming response of these systems plays the major role in causing the chronic fatigue illness, rather than being the inciting agent. After all, most people's immune system can inactivate a virus or bacteria, and they never succumb to the secondary attack by the body, which can be devastating. In one sense, CFS may be considered an autoimmune phenomenon.

The treatment for chronic fatigue syndrome in our clinic is generally focused on the immunologic imbalance as well as on brain chemistry abnormalities.

After other diseases are ruled out and a firm diagnosis of CFS is made, we spend time educating patients and encouraging them to educate themselves via the Internet and other sources. The patient that is most likely to get well is the one who takes charge of his or her own illness and becomes more educated than even his or her physician. We strongly encourage this.

Initial Treatment

I first treat the sleep problem. Sleep medications such as Elavil and Sinequan (tricyclic antidepressants) are generally useful, and CFS responds very well to Klonopin as well. While TCAs deepen and prolong sleep, Klonopin helps initiate sleep onset and down-regulates the NMDA receptor toxicity. TCAs may cause the opposite reaction of agitation in some patients. These patients usually respond well to Ambien or Sonata.

I then prescribe B12 shots at the dose of approximately 3.0 cc or 3,000 milligrams three times weekly. Some experts use even more, such as 5,000 milligrams three times weekly. One must use these heroic doses in order to fill B12 receptor sites in the central nervous system and the body.

My next approach, if the patient is not improving, is to prescribe Wellbutrin, which I believe is the most underutilized neuromodulator on the market. It can be used with any other antidepressant or antianxiety medicine with the exception of the MAOIs. It modulates both the dopamine and norepinephrine systems; therefore, it will increase concentration, energy and motivation. In many sensitive patients, one should break the tablet in half and start at 75 milligrams for approximately four days and increase to 150 milligrams for at least another week. If necessary, you can increase this to 300 milligrams, but that dose should be divided between the morning and early afternoon. This drug is not recommended for use after 4 P.M., because it can induce insomnia. When taken appropriately, the drug can actually alleviate insomnia and sleep problems, because of the normalization of the central nervous system. Always use Wellbutrin in the "SR" formulation since the short-acting tablet has increased side effects. Wellbutrin is contraindicated in the patient who has seizures, anorexia/bulimia, or uncontrolled alcoholism when seizures and DTs are possible.

Infection

If the patient has a fever and sore throat or sweats, then I am concerned that an ongoing infection is indeed occurring. There are some specific infections I am most concerned about. They include HHV-6 (human herpes virus type 6), Epstein-Barr virus, cytomegalic virus, chlamydia, mycoplasma and coagulase negative or positive staph, which can be cultured from the nose. Fortunately, most of these conditions can be treated, and I have seen remissions based upon treating these conditions.

The doses for treating HHV-6 are in the range of 500 to 750 milligrams of Famvir TID, 1,000 to 1,500 milligrams of Valtrex TID or 200 milligrams of Zovirax five times a day. One may see a response in several weeks and should continue this treatment for probably a month or longer. However, perhaps the most effective treatment is transfer factor, as described below.

If chlamydia or mycoplasma IGG and IGM titers are positive, then one should use Doxycycline 100 milligrams BID for longer than three weeks. When I use broad-spectrum antibiotics, I encourage people also to take acidophilus and probiotics to prevent yeast overgrowth syndromes. Remember that Doxycycline is a very impressive antibiotic from the standpoint of being anti-inflammatory. It down-regulates both NSFB and eosinophilic chemotactic factors, which are very powerful cytokines.[13] This, in turn, probably down-regulates TNF alpha, both in the central nervous system and in the periphery. Therefore, Doxycycline is important from two standpoints: it fights bacteria as it calms down the inflammatory storm.

If one has a coagulase positive or negative staph, one should use its sensitivities; but if there is a Methicillin resistant staph, this becomes a little bit more involved. A combination of Rifampin, Bactrim and Bactroban nasal cream applied to the nares should be used for approximately one month.

There are several other potential coinfections that should be tested for. These invaders take advantage of the immune dysregulation and do a piggyback ride into the critical systems of the body, causing more disruption in the immune and neural pathways.

A partial list of these coinfections include:

- Yeast
- Lyme—tick borne
- Babesia—tick borne
- Ehrlichiosis—tick borne
- Bacteria—harbored in the nares
- Various moles and fungi
- AIDS-type viruses

Allergy Treatment

If appropriate response is not seen after the previous steps, then my next approach is to treat the patient's overly sensitive immune response. Since most CFS patients have allergy problems, immunotherapy and neutralization have been very effective. When one reads CFS literature, this approach is rarely mentioned. This is baffling to me since the majority of CFS sufferers have inhalant allergies. My only explanation is that most allergists use the prick test, which is not sensitive enough to recognize subtle allergens seen in CFS patients. We use SET, or endpoint titration, which is more sensitive, and it also is used by the NIH for research purposes. The use of allergy shots plus a special vaccine neutralization technique have been effective in reversing the fatigue and aching of many of my CFS patients. The world-renowned Environmental Health Center in Dallas uses this as a primary approach to treat both chemical sensitivities and chronic fatigue-like syndromes.

But how does this work? I don't think anyone really knows, but this is my personal belief: It is obvious that when we treat patients with allergy shots, we are not trying to remove the allergy symptoms alone. Many CFS patients have only mild symptoms. Therefore, my purpose is not just to help allergies but also to calm a hypersensitive, overreactive immune system and thereby decrease the proinflammatory cytokines. Remember that allergy sufferers have an unusual elevation of the same inflammatory mediators that are seen in chronic fatigue syndrome. Therefore, it makes sense to treat these patients aggressively with allergy shots. It is not enough just to use oral medicines or nasal sprays. This treatment does not modify the underlying problems with the immune system, but it clearly helps.

I combine vaccine neutralization (VN) with immunotherapy as an aid to decrease the immune response. VN consists of a flu vaccine and other respiratory bacterial vaccines. We find a neutralizing dose as we test and use minute amounts of the vaccine to neutralize the body's hyper-response to viruses. This technique actually was described 50 years ago and is used by a few allergists and environmental physicians throughout the world, including the Environmental Health Center in Dallas.

Sometimes, a certain virus or another invader will induce an inflammatory response similar to an allergic phenomenon and will continue to produce symptoms even though the initial invader may have disappeared from the body. It may be this very mechanism that is the etiology of CFS. It may simply be a loco-motive that is difficult to stop once it starts. In other words, one could call it immunologic reactive inertia, that is, the inflamma-tory mediators are fighting a war when there really is no war. This is where the neutralization technique works—to calm down the body's reactivity.

CASE STUDY

A middle-aged male biochemist came to my clinic in 1995 with a 10-year history of classic CFS symptoms. He had tried virtual-ly every known therapy including herbs, vitamins and antide-pressants. He also had been to several CFS clinics. All of this was to no avail. Though he had improved mildly, he had become dis-abled and was unable to continue his career in biochemistry. His fatigue, aching, insomnia, brain fog and low-grade fevers made his quality of life extremely poor. After hearing of my approach to CFS and the success that I was having, he visited our clinic. Although his allergy symptoms were mild to moderate, we insti-tuted allergy immunotherapy and vaccine neutralization. Within approximately three months, his symptoms began to improve; and after nine months, he returned to his previous job as a biochemist. He remains in remission.

VISUAL CONTRAST TEST

To test patients for neurotoxic disease, I use the FACT, or visual contrast test. It is a simple eye test that measures the brain's ability to contrast between shades of black, gray and white. In a normal individual, this is no problem, but a patient with neurotoxic disease will not be able to differentiate the various contrasting shades. Devised by Ritchie Shoemaker, M.D., this test is a valid tool to diagnose chronic neurotoxins in the brain.[14] If a patient tests positive, the toxins need to be removed from the body, necessitating a cleansing of the system by sequestration agents as outlined below. These cellular-disrupting toxins are not easily secreted out of the body and need the help of bile resins. Bile resins grab the toxins and take them through the GI tract where they are excreted in the fecal material—this is called sequestration. It is interesting that Actos or Avandia—which helps correct insulin resistance—down-regulates TNF alpha, among other cytokines, which helps many CFS patients improve.

Actos or Avandia are given for three reasons:

1. They prevent the unwanted Jarisch-Herxheimer reaction, which is an unusual syndrome that occurs after antibiotics are given to treat an infection.
2. They reduce insulin resistance and decrease cytokine expression. This improves the underlying overreactivity of the immune system.
3. They reduce TNF alpha.

If the FACT, or visual contrast test, is positive as outlined by Dr. Shoemaker, Actos or Avandia is prescribed five days before the treatment of cholestyramine or Welchol and discontinued one to two weeks later.[15] If cholestyramine is not well tolerated, Welchol is my choice, but the improvement is much slower. A patient should continue this treatment for several months. Welchol and cholestyramine are used to trap the toxins that are traveling through the body but end up in the GI tract, wreaking havoc as they go. If they are not trapped by these medications and excreted, they will then be reabsorbed, and the vicious cycle will continue.

One of the most incredible advances in immune health in the past few years has been the development of Transfer Factors. These are tiny protein molecules called immune memory molecules, which are produced by T cells. These Factors have the amazing ability to teach the cells in the body to recognize viruses and bacteria that our bodies do not recognize. Transfer Factor is derived from colostrum, which has the important purpose to transfer immunity from the mother to her baby. Presently, colostrum can be taken from purified animal sources and is considered to be very safe. Given in medication form, Transfer Factor indeed may play a beneficial role in chronic fatigue.

VACCINE TEST/VIRAL ANTIBODY TEST

Use this vaccine/viral antibody test to check for CFS, shingles, chicken pox, flu and FMS. Prior to testing, ask the patient about present symptoms based on a scale of 1 to 10 (1 meaning free from pain and 10 meaning the worst feeling of pain). At this time, do not ask what the patient usually feels like or how he or she sometimes has felt—ask only about present symptoms.

The test itself requires an injection of .05 #2 fluogen, given intradermally. The wheal should be 7mm, firm, hard and blanched. After the shot, wait 15 to 20 minutes.

If after the waiting period the patient is relieved of all symptoms by the initial injection and the wheal is soft and no longer blanched, this is the neutralizing dose. However, if the wheal is soft and no longer blanched and the patient still has symptoms at the end of 20 minutes, inject .05 #1 dilution and wait another 15 to 20 minutes. If the wheal is still blanched and firm and remains the same size or has grown in size, and the patient still has symptoms, inject .05 #3 dilution, progressing to weaker dilutions through #6 if necessary to obtain relief. (Myalgia is the first symptom to be relieved in testing. Fever may persist until the second or third correct dose is given.)

Once the neutralizing dose has been determined, mix equal amounts of the neutralizing dose of fluogen and #3 mixed respiratory virus (MRV) in a vial. *Do not* add any diluent; only add the fluogen and #3 MRV.

Go over shot protocol (i.e., how much and how often it is to be given) and record the patient's name on your mixing calendar for two days.

Finally, get the appropriate protocol sheet and give it to the patient. The patient may receive injections in the office or take them home. Since the vaccine is safe and there is no risk of anaphylactic reaction, the patient does not have to wait and may take the vaccine home on the first day.

My Most Successful Treatments

Natural	Pharmaceuticals	Procedures
Magnesium	Wellbutrin	Allergy
Omega-3	Elavil	immunotherapy
Melatonin	Klonopin	Vaccine
3-6 milligrams		neutralization
B12 injections		
Antioxidant		
vitamins		
DHEA,		
progesterone		

CHAPTER 4

FIBROMYALGIA

Those who hope in the LORD will renew their strength. They will soar on wings like eagles; they will run and not grow weary, they will walk and not be faint.

ISAIAH 40:31

"Every morning when I wake up, I feel like I've been run over by a truck. I'm weak and sore all over." "My pain is hard to describe. I told my wife it feels like someone has pounded my whole body with a meat mallet." "It's not really a sharp or shooting pain. It's the constant feeling of aching in every cell in my body." These are descriptions of the pain felt by people suffering from fibromyalgia (FMS). "Fibro" means fibrous matter or tissue—the connective tissue that cushions joints. The suffix "-algia" means pain. "Myalgia" refers to muscle pain. The constant and severe muscle pain of fibromyalgia is what distinguishes it from the similar condition of chronic fatigue syndrome. It has been estimated that approximately 60 percent of patients with CFS also have fibromyalgia.[1]

DEFINITION

Most experts agree that fibromyalgia is not a disease but a functional disorder that causes pain in the muscles, joints, ligaments and tendons. Commonly, there are distinct points on the body that are particularly tender to the touch. They include the muscles at the base of the skull, the base of the neck, the upper back, the midback, the second rib, the side of the elbow, the upper and outer muscles of the buttocks, the upper part of the thigh and the middle of the knee.

Although fibromyalgia involves joint pain, it is not a type of arthritis or myofaciitis, which is a common muscle ache in specific areas of the body. It may be an inflammatory condition similar to rheumatism. FMS also has been known as arthralgia (pain in the joints), myalgia (pain in the muscles), fibromyositis and fibrositis, chronic muscle-contraction syndrome and psychogenic rheumatism. Over the years, attempts have been made to name and describe this condition, but it remains largely misunderstood.

Here is the story of one woman who developed FMS before it was recognized and named:

When I was in my late 30s, I started experiencing pain in all my joints, from my neck down. I went from physician to physician and had many tests run. Always, the pain continued, and the tests did not reveal the cause. I went to bed tired and got up tired. I was working full time, raising two teenage children and being a wife, which required that I had to stay up and run! Many days I hurt so bad that I couldn't remember what over-the-counter medicines I had taken.

This was before the diagnosis of FMS was even known. The doctors I went to made me feel like it was all in my head. I tried acupuncture and chiropractic, which would give me some relief for a time, but the pain would always come back. Finally my pain began to be recognized as a medical problem, and I started receiving medications to help me. Dr. Forester prescribed Effexor XR for me, and it made a great deal of difference. A regular exercise routine along with the medication has helped me tremendously. I have been retired, not disabled, for four years now. Being under stress from work was a contributing factor to the FMS. I also feel that the stress I placed upon myself was a factor in this disease. You must learn to take time daily for yourself, and if your doctor doesn't know about FMS, find one that does.[2]

SYMPTOMS

Increased sensitivity to pain is the main symptom of fibromyalgia. You may have some degree of constant pain, which can get worse depending on activity, stress, weather changes and other factors. You may have a deep ache or a burning pain, as well as muscle tightening or spasms. Much of the pain experienced by patients occurs where the muscles join the bones or tendons— particularly when the muscles are stretched. FMS symptoms generally are worst in the morning and lessen during the day. Many people have migratory pain (pain that moves around the body) that comes and goes.

Fibromyalgia does not cause permanent damage. Although your symptoms can be very uncomfortable, your muscles and organs are not being damaged. This condition is not life threatening, but it can be chronic (ongoing). However, as will be discussed later in this chapter, there are many things you can do to help you feel better. A very high percentage of my patients show great improvement when receiving proper treatment and education.

Most people with fibromyalgia feel that they have run out of energy. This fatigue may be mild or very severe. Most patients have trouble sleeping, which adds to the fatigue. They may have feelings of numbness or tingling in parts of their body, or poor circulation in some areas. Many people are very sensitive to odors, bright lights, loud noises and medicines. In addition, they may have dry eyes or difficulty focusing on nearby objects. Problems with dizziness and balance also may occur. Some people have chest pain, a rapid or irregular heartbeat or shortness of breath. Headaches and jaw pain also are common.

Digestive symptoms—difficulty swallowing, heartburn, gas, cramping abdominal pain, and alternating diarrhea and constipation—can occur with fibromyalgia. Some people have urinary complaints including frequent urination and pain in the bladder area. Women with fibromyalgia often have pelvic symptoms including painful menstrual periods and painful sexual intercourse.

Other symptoms include memory loss and mood disorders. Depression or anxiety may occur as a result of your constant pain and fatigue or the frustration you feel with the condition. It also is possible that the same chemical imbalances in the brain that cause fibromyalgia also cause depression and anxiety.

DIAGNOSIS

According to the American College of Rheumatology (ACR), to meet the criteria for a diagnosis of FMS, patients must have the following:

- Widespread pain in all four quadrants of their body for a minimum of three months
- At least 11 tender trigger points (of the 18 specified)

Key Tender (Trigger) Points of FMS

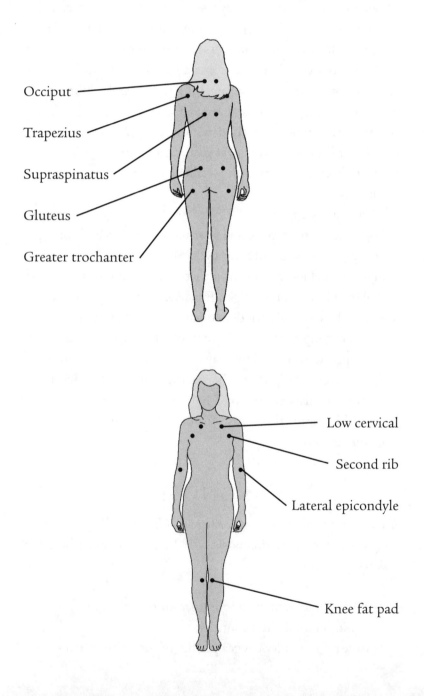

Incidence of Symptoms in FMS Patients

Symptom	Percentage of Occurrence
Pain	100 percent
Stiffness	75 to 100 percent
Subjective or objective swelling	25 to 50 percent
Fatigue	100 percent
Insomnia	50 to 75 percent
Anxiety	50 to 75 percent
Abnormal skin sensations	25 to 50 percent
Headaches	25 to 50 percent
Irritable bowel syndrome	25 to 50 percent
Depression	25 to 50 percent*

* The percentage of people having a history of depression or chronic anxiety disorders is actually less than 18 percent, but after they succumb to FMS, the incidence increases.

INCIDENCE

Of the four most common fatigue syndromes, FMS is probably second only to hypothyroidism in incidence. Two to 5 percent of all visits to primary care physicians are because of FMS. In the rheumatologist's office, the number is 6 to 20 percent. FMS is becoming a national epidemic and a major health problem, and it is time the ignorance is dispelled.[3]

According to the National Institutes of Health, approximately three to six million Americans—or 2 to 3 percent of the population—have fibromyalgia. Women of childbearing age are most likely to suffer from FMS; but children, men and the elderly also can be affected. The majority of cases begin in young adulthood. Often the symptoms begin gradually and worsen with time. Without treatment, FMS can cause major disability, as patients become unable to carry out normal activities. Here are a few encouraging words from an FMS patient who overcame these disabilities:

> My journey to "wellness" has been a journey down, through and across some of the deepest, darkest days of my life. I have faced jagged valleys that seemed to have no bottom. Is it the pain or the fatigue that causes the simplest task to become impossible? Am I losing it? What was "it" anyway?
>
> A friend tried to cheer me by commiserating, "Oh, Gwen, fibromyalgia undermines everything you are and can do—your self-esteem, self-worth and every other 'self-' that you have." That was an eye-opener, or should I say tear-starter. I promptly left the party to walk outside, bawl and talk with God! I realized that FMS had undermined my relationship with my husband, family and God. It has restricted my ability to work with and minister to the hearing impaired. Everything important to me was being sucked down into the dark cracks along with my health. I realized that my life could not go on in this way and, yes, even the darkest thoughts of suicide crossed my mind.
>
> Dr. Forester helped bring light into my darkness. I have been seeing him for FMS and chronic fatigue for several years and have experienced success with many different combinations of therapy. However, on one special day, I asked him to pray for me. He immediately laid his hand on my shoulder and prayed for me. He then gave me a word from God—"You are special!" He didn't know that I felt worthless due to my health, but God

used him to begin a healing of my spirit, mind and body! I am now closer to being "pain-free" than I have been in years. The combination of Effexor, magnesium, Vivactil and Guaifenesin have given me hope for today—I can do it! (As soon as I remember what "it" is, and where I put "it"!) Humor is a great medicine!

I want to encourage all my FMS friends: keep your smile, keep your supports, and find a caring physician who understands the complexity and craziness of FMS.[4]

CAUSES

Most experts today believe that FMS is caused by a biologic response to physical or emotional stress in certain individuals who are susceptible because of genetic factors or past trauma or both. The most common triggers in the onset of the disorder seem to be major accidents or injuries, especially upper spine injury, accumulated minor trauma, viral or bacterial infections and chronic stress.

Fibromyalgia was once thought to be depression, anxiety or a psychosomatic illness. Some clinicians would laugh and call the sufferers, "Oh, those 'emotional' women." After all, there was no verifiable blood test or X ray that could prove that FMS had an organic basis. However, in the past two decades, knowledge about brain chemistry and inflammatory mediators has grown tremendously. We now know that FMS is quite clearly an abnormality in the neurochemistry of the central nervous system, which in turn affects the endocrine system.[5]

More recently, FMS was thought to be an arthritic-type disease, so doctors referred patients to rheumatologists, who then assumed the treatment of this syndrome. Rheumatologists do well in helping rheumatoid arthritis, lupus, Sjorgren's and the like, but their expertise is not in dealing with the central nervous system. The burden was placed on rheumatologists to treat these poor sufferers with the same medicines used to treat rheumatoid arthritis. They did, in the beginning, discover that small doses of Elavil (a tricyclic antidepressant) at night seemed to help their patients, which was interpreted early on that FMS was simply depression. But there was a contradiction. Doses of Elavil that proved effective for FMS were much lower than those needed for depression. Nevertheless, the rheumatologists sort of acquiesced to the burden of treating what appeared to be an arthritis-like syndrome. The science of the twenty-first century has proven that *it is not.*[6]

As stated previously, one current belief is that FMS is triggered by an injury or emotional trauma that may affect the nervous system. Others believe a virus is responsible, but no specific infectious agent has been identified. The National Institute of Arthritis and Musculoskeletal and Skin Diseases (NIAMS) is currently using post-Lyme Disease syndrome as a model for research since many patients develop FMS-like symptoms following Lyme disease. They also are conducting studies to examine the interaction between the nervous system and the endocrine system, and the regulation of adrenal function in FMS patients. Low levels of cortisol, a hormone produced by the adrenal glands, may be associated with FMS. In addition, research involving patients' levels of growth hormone is underway. Since growth hormone is produced during sleep, patients may be deficient because of the sleep disturbance common in FMS.[7]

A common pain-inducing factor in FMS is that of physical injury, especially to a nerve or set of nerves. In one study, fibromyalgia developed in over 20 percent of patients who had neck injuries. Pain may result from a ruptured disc, spinal stenosis (narrowing in the spinal canal), thoracic outlet syndrome (narrowing where the nerves exit from the first rib), neuropathy or neuritis (a "sick nerve"). These are a few instances in which a nerve is the source of the pain, and this is called neuropathic pain. It is important to be tested for spine or nerve irregularities, especially if your FMS began after a car accident or other type of major injury or surgery.

Sitting in front of a computer every day for years can be another form of injury. Cumulative minor stresses on your spinal column, neck and back can result from weakened and sedentary muscles, bad posture and tension. Being in a frozen position for many hours at a time is not likely to be a cause of FMS, but it can be a contributing factor and needs to be considered in an overall treatment plan.

I have come to believe, along with many other practitioners and researchers, that fibromyalgia is not a muscle illness; rather, it is a central nervous system illness caused by abnormalities in the brain and spinal cord.

Through years of experience treating fibromyalgia, I have come to believe, along with many other practitioners and researchers, that it is not a muscle illness; rather, it is a central nervous system illness caused by abnormalities in the brain and spinal cord. This is illustrated when researchers have measured certain chemicals in the spinal fluid of FMS patients and found proinflammatory cytokines elevated as much as four-fold.[8] Specific types of cytokines such as substance P, nerve growth factor and tumor necrosis factor-alpha appear to be vital in the pathophysiology of this illness. Neurotransmitters such as norepinephrine and serotonin are low in the spinal fluid, thus implicating these substances in the process as well.[9] Let me add that one does not see these inflammatory cytokines elevated in depression or anxiety, which some clinicians still believe is at the heart of FMS. Depression is not a risk factor in the development of FMS, but in

FMS patients, depression is common. It appears secondary to the process.

A Short Course in Neurology

The last 10 or so years have been called the decade of the brain. Some amazing facts have been discovered, and the intricate workings of the brain and nervous system have been the subject of numerous books and articles. We know the nervous system contains an incredible network of minicomputers with an astounding array of connections, chemicals and cells.

The central nervous system is comprised of the brain and spinal cord. All the nerves that branch out and penetrate the rest of the body are called the peripheral nervous system. The nervous system can be divided into two components: the autonomic (or involuntary) system and the somatic (or voluntary) system. The autonomic system is very complex, controlling most bodily functions not under conscious control, such as blood pressure, heart rate, hormone secretion and so on. The somatic system controls actions that are voluntary, sending messages from the brain to muscles that enable us to walk, talk and so on.

Autonomic Nervous System	Somatic Nervous System
Heart action	Sense organs
Breathing	Voluntary muscles
Sweating	Any actions and activities
Pupil dilation	under your control
Sleep/Wakefulness	

The autonomic system contains two divisions: the parasympathetic (PNS) and the sympathetic (SNS). The SNS is the "accelerator," and it keeps our heart beating, our stomach and intestines digesting, our bladder contracting and so on. Even during sleep, these and other vital functions are kept going. The SNS is responsible for defensive and offensive activities for survival. It has been called the fight, fright and flight system. Adrenaline and noradrenaline are its primary chemical mediators. The PNS is the "brake" of the system. It slows the heart rate, lowers blood pressure and induces sleep. When the PNS is activated, the blood is flooded with acetycholine, a chemical that helps relax the system. One may think of the SNS as being most active during the day—to energize us to move, think and react. The PNS rules at bedtime—to calm us and keep vital functions going while restorative activities silently take place during sleep.

The sympathetic and parasympathetic nervous systems are constantly working in tandem to keep the body in balance. Neither one is ever in complete control, but they complement each other to keep the body's functions fine-tuned. An imbalance in this mechanism is called dysautonomia. In FMS, there is evidence that dysautonomia occurs.[10] The SNS is overactivated at night, disallowing appropriate, restful sleep. The PNS is overactive during the day, producing fatigue, brain fog and sedation. Research is in progress to find an SNS blocker to help turn off the nighttime activation. Hopefully, this medication will be able to help with the disturbed sleep of FMS and allow the patient to enter the deeper stages of sleep hindered in these individuals.

Dysautonomia symptoms in FMS include the following:

- Enhanced pain sensitivity
- Increased muscle tension, pain at rest
- Numbness and tingling sensations
- Disturbed sleep

- Brain fog—"wired but tired" leads to trouble concentrating
- Migraine headaches
- Dry eyes and mouth
- GI symptoms—indigestion and abdominal cramping
- Urinary urgency
- Fatigue—exhausted all the time
- Low blood pressure
- Dizziness
- Faintness
- Shortness of breath
- Cold, clammy hands
- Difficulty relaxing
- Cold intolerance—unable to respond well to drafts and rapid weather changes

BRAIN PAIN

In FMS patients, dysfunction seems to exist in the somatic as well as the autonomic nervous system. This involves the pain pathways. Because it has been demonstrated that fibromyalgia is not characterized by abnormalities in the muscles, you may think, *Why do my muscles hurt when there is no obvious physical cause? Is it in my head?* Well, *it is in your head*. Let me explain.

Pain is a sensation. It is felt in the body but perceived and interpreted in the brain. The physical sensation of pain contains three components:

1. Peripheral—where the pain occurs in the body
2. Spinal cord—where the signal is processed and transmitted
3. Brain—the final command and control center where interpretation of the pain is perceived, modulated and interpreted

In FMS, the pain input is misinterpreted by the brain and felt to a heightened level. Pain experts call this allodynia. Allodynia, the scourge of FMS sufferers, is the perception of pain from stimuli that do not ordinarily cause pain. Therefore, the pain may not really be painful to healthy people, but it debilitates FMS sufferers.[11] Why does this happen?

Most people have heard of the three major neurotransmitters, or brain chemicals—serotonin (SE), dopamine (DA) and norepinephrine (NE)—which are contained in the synapses of the brain cells. These play a major role in controlling mood and behavior as well as other functions such as pain perception. For example, if the amount of serotonin is decreased in the brain, depression, anxiety, migraine headaches and insomnia can result. If one has low levels of norepinephrine, depression, low energy and low concentration are experienced. Low dopamine in the synaptic gaps of the brain will result in a lack of sexual function and pleasure in life, low motivation and addictive tendencies.

One may look at these chemicals as modulators, similar to a powerful dimmer switch. Essentially, they are the fine tuners of how we feel and think. They modify the fatigue and pain response of the body. If these master chemicals are altered in the smallest amount, one can experience major changes in emotional or physical symptoms.

Neurophysiologists use the words "down-regulate" when referring to turning down the dimmer switch, thereby decreasing brain chemical activity. A complex array of inhibitory fibers and synapses are involved in down regulation. "Up-regulate" means to turn up the dimmer switch to produce a greater and more intense firing of nerve cells. We use medicines today either to down-regulate or to up-regulate nerve cell systems, thereby decreasing or increasing the perception of pain. SSRIs (selective serotonin reuptake inhibitors) and TCAs (tricyclic antidepressants) are commonly prescribed for FMS patients to help in regulating the delicate balance of brain chemicals.

TREATMENTS

FMS treatment is not complicated once one realizes that the basis of the pain is in the brain and not in the body. It is clearly neuropathic, which means one has a malfunctioning nervous system. This is different—as stated above—than somatic pain, which involves joints, soft tissues and bone. Coexisting conditions do exist, of course, such as arthritis, irritable bowel syndrome and myofasciitis, but the component that must be addressed is clearly neurological. The four major parameters relating to this, as outlined by Dr. Paul Cheney, a pioneer in the treatment of CFS and FMS, are the following:

- Sleep
- Myalgia, or pain
- Fatigue
- Cerebral[12]

At our clinic, we use these four major symptoms as benchmarks of how severe the condition is and how effective the treatment is. Almost all of my patients show a high degree of recovery in these four areas.

Drug Treatments

The first step is to modulate the serotonin and norepinephrine brain chemicals and to address insomnia. This step can be achieved by starting a patient on a tricyclic antidepressant (TCA) such as Elavil (amitriptyline). TCAs are older antidepressants seldom used today for depression due to their side effects, but in lower doses they are very effective for sleep improvement and reduction of chronic pain. I believe Elavil is the best because it helps level out the balance of serotonin and norepinephrine better than any other tricyclic. TCAs are excellent for FMS, because they enhance the deepening of sleep, improve the disturbance of altered sleep architecture, relax muscles, decrease depression and modulate the secretion of pain-relieving endorphins. The downside of these medicines is that they can produce weight gain, cause hangover and occasionally produce constipation, agitation and/or hypertension. However, since many FMS sufferers require only low doses, the mentioned side effects are less common; and in my practice, tricyclics are very well tolerated. If Elavil is not effective in reducing symptoms, an antidepressant called Effexor can also be added for rebalancing brain chemicals. Effexor appears to be more effective than the more common SSRIs such as Prozac and Zoloft because of its greater impact on norepinephrine levels. If Elavil causes hangover, Tofranil is recommended.

The hormones DHEA and progesterone both up-regulate dopamine and help modulate cortisol production, which helps some FMS patients. They are best metabolized in transdermal form, and creams are available from compounding pharmacies.

Many FMS patients are hesitant to try any medications because they know their bodies are extra sensitive, and they may have had bad reactions to drugs in the past. However, some patients also feel desperate—like they have reached the bottom of the bucket. They have no reserves left and need a remedy to get them started on the road to being well. Let me try to reassure patients about drug treatment, should a physician suggest it. Drugs can work like a cast that will temporarily support people as their body is getting better. It's as if their brain is broken and they need to do something to prop it up during the healing process. The drugs do not heal them any more than a cast heals a broken leg. Drugs provide support and allow people's bodies to begin the process of strengthening itself. Then the patient will slowly be able to discontinue the medications.

Even when medications are having a positive effect on an illness, they are no substitute for stress reduction, exercise or other necessary lifestyle changes. They are seldom the long-term solution. Making healthy choices will help patients get better and *stay* well after they have tapered off any drugs they may have taken.

Emotional and Mental Component

As with any chronic illness, emotional problems can worsen the condition and may be a contributing factor to triggering FMS. Ask God to help you recognize and understand the mental stresses in your life. Negative emotions such as anger, anxiety and resentment can actually change the chemistry of the brain, making an individual more susceptible to nervous system dysfunction. Physical pain can feel worse when you are experiencing emotional conflict.

Anxiety is a harmful emotion for many reasons. Anxiety and worry only worsen the disease process by dampening the immune response and even raising cytokine production. Anxiety is the number one cause for insomnia, and sleep difficulties exacerbate any condition. Anxiety decreases self-control and can lead to overeating, drinking alcohol and smoking. It elevates blood pressure, worsens acid reflux and contributes to heart disease. Therefore, it is important to remember this key biblical verse when dealing with anxiety:

[Never be anxious ever (from the Greek)], but in everything, by prayer and petition, with thanksgiving, present
your requests to God. And the peace of God, which tran-
scends all understanding, will guard your hearts and
your minds in Christ Jesus (Phil. 4:6-7).

If you have unresolved conflicts or bitterness toward your spouse, parent, boss or coworker, your body is being harmed. If you are a high-achieving workaholic who is always in a hurry and has too much to do, damage may be occurring to your nervous system. If you are nagged with continual worries and fears, your physical well-being is at risk. While medications, diet and exercise are major components in regaining your health, forgiveness, anger management and letting go of controlling, perfectionist tendencies are equally vital. These words Paul wrote to the Ephesians are a blueprint for optimal mental health:

While medications, diet and exercise are major components in regaining your health, forgiveness, anger management and letting go of controlling, perfectionist tendencies are equally vital.

> Get rid of all bitterness, rage and anger, brawling and slander, along with every form of malice. Be kind and compassionate to one another, forgiving each other, just as in Christ God forgave you (Eph. 4:31-32).

Exercise

Exercise promotes sleep and decreases pain and tenderness by helping to keep brain chemicals in balance. Our bodies are designed to be active. However, many FMS patients have become deconditioned because intense activity can make them feel worse. The key is graded exercise—start very slowly and gradually build up strength and endurance. Even though your muscles hurt, the muscles still need to move to stay fit. One of the best things you can do is low-impact aerobic exercise. Examples of this type of exercise include swimming or water exercise, stationary bicycling and walking on a level surface. You may need to begin at a very low level of exercise (maybe just five minutes every other day). The day after you exercise, you might feel worse. But don't get discouraged. Keep at it. Continue to increase the length and frequency of activity until you are exercising for 30 minutes at least four times a week. Once you reach this point, you can consider switching to high-impact exercises like jogging and tennis. Also, light massage after exercise can reduce muscle aches and speed up recovery time.

Aquatic therapy (or hydrotherapy) is especially helpful and is best done in water that is around 85 degrees Fahrenheit for 15 to 30 minutes at a time, two or three times a week. Many YMCAs have warm-water therapy pools and offer low-energy classes. Water therapy should include walking, stretching and water-resistance exercises. Being immersed in water that is somewhat cooler than your body temperature causes your body core to cool, resulting in a decrease in proinflammatory cytokines. When standing in water, the increased pressure in your feet and legs causes a squeezing action in the lymph system. This forces lymph fluid into the bloodstream, signaling your body that enough cytokines are circulating, which results in a lessening of inflammation and pain.

Stretching is important for maintaining flexibility and loosening painfully tight muscles. Make it a daily priority to gently stretch neck, back and leg muscles. Your physician or physical therapist can teach you specific stretching exercises that are appropriate for FMS patients.

Diet

Proper nutrition is a key ingredient of well-being, especially for those with low energy levels and chronic illness. To perform at maximum efficiency, the body needs foods that are nutrient-dense. Snacks and fast foods that are filled with sugar, fat, caffeine, salt, additives and flavorings will not provide proper fuel for the body. High-fat diets have been shown to worsen fibro-cystic breast disease and multiple sclerosis, and they may also have a negative effect on fibromyalgia. Saturated fats contained in dairy products, meat and margarine can interfere with circu-lation, increasing inflammation and pain. Trans fats, which result from frying foods in hydrogenated vegetable oils, actually change the structure of brain cell membranes, which can dimin-ish mental performance.

Sugar and caffeine are stimulants, as powerful as any drug. Every time you eat a sugary snack or drink coffee or soda, a boost in adrenaline occurs, followed by a letdown. The FMS patient's autonomic nervous system is extremely sensitive to this roller-coaster effect of sugar and caffeine. Caffeine has a strong affect on brain biochemistry—mainly dopamine receptors. It raises blood pressure, interferes with REM sleep cycles and ele-vates the body's reaction to stress. Remember that chocolate also contains high amounts of sugar and caffeine. Some medications contain caffeine, so it is wise to read labels carefully. Alcohol—in addition to sugar and caffeine—can enhance fatigue, increase muscle pain and interfere with normal sleep patterns.

FMS patients should avoid the following "excite toxins," meaning that they have a toxic effect on brain chemistry.

- Sugar
- Caffeine (soft drinks, coffee, black tea, chocolate, cer-tain medications and so on)
- Alcohol
- Tobacco
- Saturated fats (fatty meats, cheese, margarine, fried foods and so on)
- Processed foods (most contain sugar, preservatives, additives and/or hydrogenated fats)
- NutraSweet and MSG

A healthy diet for an FMS patient is based on consuming foods as close to their natural state as possible. This includes plenty of raw and steamed vegetables, lean meats and fish, nuts, fruits and whole grains. Choose brown rice over white rice and whole wheat bread over white bread for their nutrient density and fiber content. Eating five or six small meals a day will help keep your energy level even by lessening the effects of blood-sugar changes. Many of my patients find they feel better when they eat a healthy snack every hour or two. Drinking six to eight glasses of water each day helps to keep your body sufficiently hydrated and is important for flushing out toxins. Herbal teas and fruit juices are good substitutes for coffee and soft drinks.

A healthy diet for an FMS patient is based on consuming foods as close to their natural state as possible.

Herbs and Vitamins

Herbal agents are touted by some to be FMS healing agents, but none of my patients have demonstrated any sustained improvement in either CFS or FMS with herbs.

Antioxidants help reduce free-radical damage and fight inflammation. Therefore, I encourage my patients to take minerals and vitamins, especially the antioxidants vitamins E, A and C, as well as zinc and magnesium. Optimum doses are 5,000 to 10,000 international units of vitamin A per day, 400 to 800 international units of vitamin E per day and 2,000 to 4,000 milligrams of vitamin C per day. Coenzyme Q-10 also is an antioxidant and can be beneficial in doses of 60 milligrams twice daily. Folic acid and B vitamins are vital but probably not curative in and of themselves.

The most effective supplement for lessening the symptoms of CFS are the essential fatty acids (EFAs). They are important in cell-wall function in the 55 trillion cells of the body—especially the brain. Our Western diet is deficient in omega-3 fatty acids, and they cannot be manufactured by the body. Since very few foods consumed in our diet contain these EFAs, supplements are particularly beneficial.

Physical Therapies

Some patients have been helped by treatments such as physical therapy, chiropractic adjustment and massage. All muscles are surrounded by myofascial connective tissues. These tissues play an important role in the stretching and contracting of the muscles as well as providing pathways for nerves and blood vessels. In FMS, myofascial tissues contract due to neurotransmitter disturbances, which in turn cause compression of nerves and vessels. This constant tension and inflammation contributes to pain and tenderness. Using massage with passive stretching techniques can release myofascial tissue and significantly reduce muscle tension. Massage also increases blood supply to the tissue, which transports more oxygen and nutrients, as well as removes toxic buildup by stimulating lymph drainage. Choose a massage therapist or nonforce chiropractor who is experienced in working with FMS patients and can provide a gentle, therapeutic touch that is not overly aggressive.

Lifestyle Adaptation

Much improvement can be realized by understanding what makes your symptoms worse and adjusting your life to accommodate those factors. Because fibromyalgia symptoms are worsened by stress and poor sleep, it is crucial to decrease the stresses in your life whenever possible and to get as much rest as you need. Other simple lifestyle changes may be helpful. For example, try keeping your activity level the same each day. Many people with fibromyalgia try to do as much as possible on good days, which leads them to have several bad days. Keeping your activity level consistent may decrease the number of bad days.

The people with whom you surround yourself can be beneficial to your condition or can add to your stress level. "Toxic" relationships are not healthy. Choose to spend time with friends who are positive, upbeat and encouraging and who make you laugh. Avoid people who drag you down with their complaining, negative or bossy attitudes. Some people are high-maintenance energy-drainers and are exhausting just to be around. Others, with their good humor and healthy outlook, can help you forget about how bad you feel.

Most FMS patients are extrasensitive to changes in weather. Therefore, it's a good idea to stay in environments that are as constant as possible. One patient said, "When it's 75 degrees and clear, with no wind, I feel pretty good! But the minute the air pressure or temperature changes, my symptoms kick in. On cold, rainy days, I ache all over and feel like my body weighs about 500 pounds. I can barely move. When a dry east wind blows, I get terrible headaches and stiffness. I feel like a giant barometer!" Cold, wet climates especially seem to worsen pain in FMS patients, and heat increases fatigue. Don't expose yourself to low temperatures by spending time outdoors in the winter. You may need to bundle up more than most people to keep your body comfortable when it's cold. In extreme heat, keep your activity level to a minimum. Some people with FMS have gone to the extreme of relocating to an area with a moderate climate for the sake of their health.

Attitude

Being constantly tired and in pain can cause anyone's outlook on life to deteriorate. People who were once optimistic and cheerful often become discouraged and fearful. Trying to have a good attitude seems impossible. However, any amount of

thankfulness, hope and humor you can muster will contribute
to your well-being:

A cheerful heart is good medicine, but a crushed spirit
dries up the bones (Prov. 17:22).

You are probably mourning the loss of your former capabilities. You miss many activities that used to give you pleasure and
purpose. It's important to acknowledge your loss and allow yourself to feel the sadness, but then move on. Instead of dwelling on
the things you can't do anymore, think about what you *can* do.
Cultivate some new interests and hobbies while you're regaining
your health. One patient who could no longer continue to sing in
her church's praise band or participate in active sports decided to
try a new creative outlet—sculpture. It didn't take much energy,
and it gave her something new on which to focus. You might try
some of the following tips from patients:

- Read about something new—order books online that
  cover subjects with which you're unfamiliar.
- Watch humorous videos.
- Write encouraging notes to people who also are ill.
- Attempt unique, low-energy forms of exercise like
  aquatic stretching.

Quilt, garden, play Jeopardy on the computer or take out
that musical instrument you haven't picked up in years.
Basically, you want to keep your mind and body as active as possible, which will help divert your attention away from your
health problems.

The key to having a "cheerful heart" is not to give in to discouragement and fear. If you ask Him, God will give you a heart
of gratitude and hopefulness in the midst of your suffering.

He wants you to be well and will guide you in your path to healing. David told his son Solomon:

> Do not be afraid or discouraged, for the LORD God, my
> God, is with you. He will not fail you or forsake you
> (1 Chron. 28:20).

You can hold on to that promise just as Solomon did during his weakest moments.

I'll end this particular section with a short anecdote by a patient, who attempts to see the humorous side of her FMS condition.

"Secondary" Symptoms of Fibromyalgia

Anyone with fibromyalgia knows that this condition has numerous symptoms that are common within the FMS population. However, after living with FMS for a while, you also may become familiar with the "secondary" symptoms. If you do, know that you are not alone.

Acute Pain: Most often caused by accidental encounters with doorjambs, walls and stair steps, it also can be caused by slamming body parts into household appliances, drawers or vehicle doors.

Pseudovertigo: This is not really about dizziness, but instead it is the tendency to suddenly list, lean or even fall sideways when you were previously standing still.

Social Fumble: Normally occurring when you are really fatigued and should have been in bed hours ago, this symptom can manifest itself by causing you to call people by any name other than their own, carry on a conversation without making any sense whatsoever and to completely forget every noun that you ever knew.

Out-of-Body Experience: Not to be confused with daydreaming, and sometimes described as "lost time," this is actually a form of "fibro fog." It normally occurs when you are reading, watching TV or trying to answer e-mail. With your brain at maximum overload, it actually stops to download, leaving the shell of your body frozen in sit-and-stare mode for 10-30 minutes.

Misplacement: This is a frequently occurring symptom and actually has an up side. It can be good physical and mental exercise. This symptom involves the PWFMS (person with FMS) putting an item somewhere and then forgetting where that somewhere is. The item can be as small as a fork or as large as a car. This symptom knows no boundaries as it can happen at home, at work or at any public place.

Radical Reactivity: A true fibro art form. This symptom relies on external stimulus. Stimuli can be divided into two categories: personal or chemical. The chemical stimulus can be as innocent as skin lotion or a whiff of your local department store perfume counter. Reactivity can range from allergic reaction to migraine. Personal stimulus involves another person quietly entering a room, therefore startling the PWFMS, causing a severe CNS reaction that escalates to a physical reaction (i.e., jumping out of your skin and up toward the ceiling) and/or an audible reaction (i.e., loosely translated as EEEEHHHUUGGGHHHH).[13]

CONCLUSION

1. There is a growing epidemic of FMS in Western countries.

2. The biochemical abnormality is in the brain and not the muscles.
3. Depression is not a common precursor but sometimes occurs secondarily.
4. Appropriate medications and supplements can help balance the central nervous system, which relieves the pain peripherally.
5. One must eat right, exercise and sleep well to improve.
6. It is vital to resolve any mental and emotional factors, such as conflict and resentment.
7. Making changes in your life to avoid stress is essential.

TO THE PHYSICIAN

FIBROMYALGIA

Epidemiology	Estimated 2 to 3% of population
Key symptoms and history	1. Generally slow onset
	2. Chronic fatigue
	3. Aching, tender muscles
	4. Unrestful sleep, insomnia
	5. Brain fog
Diagnosis	Simple and straighforward
Treatment approach	1. Moderately difficult
	2. Side effects to drugs can be unusual

Continued on next page

Continued from previous page

| **Prognosis** | 1. Poor if not diagnosed or treated wisely
2. Spontaneous remission uncommon
3. Improvement or remission possible for majority of patients |

In fibromyalgia, the important modulators norepinephrine and serotonin are decreased, and when they are at low levels in the brain, pain is interpreted at a higher level. It appears that proinflammatory cytokines (as described earlier) are producing a "fire" in the nervous system to the point that allodynia rather than authentic pain is a culprit. The chemical and neural abnormalities found in FMS patients cause the brain to become hypersensitive, and therefore a physician must address the brain abnormality and not treat it as a body abnormality. In FMS, the body chemistries are basically normal, the muscles and connective tissue are normal, and the bursal and tendon processes are basically normal. The abnormality clearly exists in the central nervous system. Therefore, why do physicians continue to treat the illness with Tylenol, Advil, Naprosyn or Cortisone? Or why do they treat it just as depression?

CASE STUDY

A 57-year-old woman came into my clinic in early 2002. She had suffered from fibromyalgia for approximately 10 years, having gone from one physician to another without any improvement. She heard about my clinic and made an appointment. Her story is typical of what we hear. Her fibromyalgia was one of slow onset—progressive—that eventually produced insomnia, pain in muscles, brain fog and eventually depression. She was taking Zoloft, NSAIDS and sleep medicine. Her quality of life was extremely poor. After hearing her story, I gave her hope. I told her that we could get her better by improving the chemical balance in her brain and decreasing the inflammation in her nerves. We started her on Effexor and Elavil and stopped the other medicines. We augmented her sleep with Ambien. She returned in one month in virtual remission from this 10-year scourge. She was literally amazed that a few simple changes in medication could make such a big difference.

SCIENTIFIC CONCEPTS AND DEFINITION

When one reads FMS literature, one very seldom finds a definition of FMS. Articles usually say, "FMS is characterized by . . . ," but they never offer a true definition. This is my FMS definition, and it is consistent with the knowledgeable literature of today:

> FMS is a stress-induced, maladaptive disorder of the CNS involving compromised neuroplasticity causing central sensitization, up-regulated cytokine expression and neuroendocrine pathology, resulting in allodynia, chronic fatigue and unrestful sleep.

It is possible to add to this definition, because FMS is very complicated, but the sentence above is the crux of the matter. Now let's break it down and look at the various components:

1. Some types of stress to the genetically susceptible individual can induce FMS. FMS literature has docu-

mented several identifiable risk factors that include early childhood stress or abuse, chronic (ongoing) stress, injury (especially to the CNS), infections, type II axis disorders and unresolved anger accompanied by a compulsive personality.

2. Neuroplasticity is a new concept in medicine, defined first by Michael Merzenich, a California otologist. What we have realized today is that chronic conditions of the brain such as lifelong depression, anxiety and FMS exhibit compromised neuroplasticity, which is the remarkable "capacity of the nervous system to adapt or modify to imposed change."[14] This means that the brain is able to add new neural pathways and break down others, depending upon experience.

3. Central sensitization is defined as an exaggerated pathological response to a stimulus that was originally innocuous. Perhaps the central core of FMS is NMDA up-regulation in the spinal cord, which greatly amplifies painless stimuli into pain. Essentially, the brain deceives itself. To make things worse, the descending inhibitory pathways that normally quell pain are malfunctioning. These pathways have two sources: One is in the raphe nucleus, and the other originates in the locus coerulus, which are innervated by serotonin and norepinephrine, respectively. (This explains why Effexor XR and TCAs are so effective.) In FMS, these pathways are ineffective in subduing the pain response. Therefore, a vicious cycle of pain results.

4. Up-regulated cytokines in the spinal fluid include substance P, nerve growth factor, interleukin 1 and interleukin 6. The blocking of interleukin 6 relieves pain and brain fog in FMS patients. Neuroscientists

Watkins and Meier believe that these immune mediators are the major cause of pain. Their colleague, Erin
Milligan, Ph.D., stated in a 2002 American Pain
Society meeting that one injection of IL-1 receptor
antagonist (IL1-1ra) quickly resolves allodynia in animal models. These studies are very exciting, since new
medications can be developed based upon this
research. Remember that allodynia simply means that
nonpainful stimuli are perceived as painful. This is
the hallmark symptom of FMS.

Another aspect of this exaggerated immune
response was described at a 2003 meeting of the
LAFP, where I also was a speaker. Patrick Wood, M.D.,
professor of family medicine and psycopharmacology
at LSU Medical Center in Shreveport, reported that
FMS patients had exaggerated mast cell reactivity.
This was associated with irritable bowel syndrome
(IBS), food sensitivities (and allergies), inhalant allergies and interstitial cystitis. This explains some of the
co-morbidities in FMS patients.

5. Insomnia may be due to abnormal alpha-delta waves,
   which suppress normal stage 3 and 4 sleep. This also
   is seen in other chronic pain states. Dr. Wood believes
   this represents the hypervigilant stress response of
   the brain. In other words, stress has taught the brain
   to accommodate light, nonrestorative sleep. And
   since sleep is the "caretaker of the brain" (in my definition), the brain is not being cared for in FMS. This
   is another aspect of the vicious cycle. Remember,
   TCAs remove these interfering alpha-delta waves and
   allow the patient to experience stage 3 and stage 4
   sleep.

6. It has been documented that chronic stress induces

elevated cortisol due to up-regulated CRF (corticotropin-releasing factor) and CRH (corticotropin-releasing hormone) released by the hypothalamus and pituitary, respectively. At the same time, the hippocampus and amygdala are both disregulated. The hippocampus is vital to learning and memory, and it is the modulation of the stress response. In FMS, it becomes somewhat atrophied and cannot inhibit the stress cycle. On the other hand, the amygdala is abnormally up-regulated and sends messages of fear and anxiety to many parts of the brain. These processes contribute to the exaggerated NMDA (N-methyl D-aspartate) response to pain.

7. A common pathway of fatigue is found in the mitochondrial mechanisms. *It has been discovered that of all of the cellular organelles, these energy factories are the most susceptible to oxidant injury.* We know that the chronic stress response depletes important electron scavengers such as glutathione—the important protector of mitochondial and cellular mechanisms. Incidentally, glutathione can be depleted by low-dose chronic mercury intoxication. Therefore, glutathione repletion is vital. Other important antioxidants are listed in the upcoming treatment section.

These pathologic mechanisms have been simplified and summarized for the sake of time and space. FMS is a very complicated syndrome, and extensive information can be found in medical and scientific literature. More maladaptive mechanisms are known, too. The ones described above, I believe, represent the essentials. In understanding these principles, one can formulate a viable treatment plan.

DIAGNOSIS

Refer back to page 80 to revisit the key tender (trigger) points of FMS. Additionally, please reread the "Symptoms" and "Diagnosis" sections at the beginning of this chapter. The follwing diagram describes various body reactions of FMS patients.

Body Reactions of FMS Patients

Musculoskeletal
   Trigger point sites 2 . . . to allodynia

Endocrine
   Low overall production of cortisol
   Low growth hormone secretion
   Hypothalamic/pituitary axis dysfunction
   Dysautonomia (at rest, hyperactive sympathetic nervous
      system; activity-induced hypoactive nervous system)

Central Nervous System
   Low serotonin and norepinephrine
   Elevated substance P
   Elevated nerve growth factor
   Elevated calcitonin gene–related peptide
   Elevated dynorphin A
   Low dopamine

Sleep
   Alpha-wave intrusion of delta sleep activity
   Impairment of stage 3 and 4 non-REM sleep correlating
      with nonrestorative sleep

Continued from previous page

Cardiovascular
Prevalence of neurally mediated hypotension during tilt-table testing

TREATMENT

My drug treatment of FMS patients usually begins with the TCA Elavil. The usual starting dose is 10 milligrams unless by history one discovers that the patient is very sensitive to medications, in which case I will start at 5 milligrams. (If a patient is overly sensitive to caffeine and alcohol, you can almost always assume that he or she will also be sensitive to any medication that affects the nervous system.) I generally increase the dose about every third or fourth night by 10 milligrams until sleep is restored and the patient's pain is being relieved.

Amitriptyline also is very effective for sleep and has been shown to stabilize sleep/wake homeostasis. Some physicians prefer imipramine, which may achieve the same results without increased sedation. Patients should take the TCA approximately two hours before bedtime for two reasons:

1. The onset of sleep is rather slow.
2. There is a decrease in the hangover effect the next day.

If the patient is unable to tolerate a TCA, Zanaflex, an A-2 receptor blocker, is an excellent alternative. Zanaflex is termed a muscle relaxant, but it has a central nervous system action that diminishes pain by modulating the norepinephrine system. It can be used for sleep at a two- to four-milligram dose; and that dose can be repeated approximately three to four hours later—in the middle of the night, if necessary. Neurontin also helps sleep and pain. I start in low doses of 100 milligrams and increase to 600 milligrams at bedtime. If a patient generally is not sensitive to medicines, 300 milligrams can be the starting dose.

Effexor

If the Elavil does not resolve pain and sleep problems, I always prescribe Effexor because of its enhanced effect on norepinephrine levels. SSRIs such as Prozac, Zoloft, Celexa and Luvox are generally ineffective. We do see many patients coming to our office having been placed on SSRIs such as Prozac and Zoloft. These antidepressants do not significantly involve the norepinephrine system (with the exception of higher doses of Paxil) and seem to be ineffective in FMS patients.

Again, the treatment of pain is aimed at modifying the chemistry and the inflammation of the central nervous system. In my opinion, the number one drug of choice for the pain and fatigue of FMS is Effexor XR. However, it must be given at appropriate dosage levels to improve both SE and NE balance. One should begin at 37.5 milligrams for the first week, increase it to 75 milligrams for the second week, and by the third week, one should be taking the 150-milligram tablet. After approximately two to four weeks of the 150-milligram dose, one should increase to 225 milligrams if no improvement in pain and fatigue or sleep occur.

Let me emphasize that the dose of at least 150 milligrams is needed in order to up-regulate the serotonin and norepinephrine systems. This is very important since we know that neuropathic pain responds to higher doses of Effexor.[15] I believe that these doses significantly down-regulate the pain-inducing cytokines, substance P and nerve growth factor. If Effexor is not tolerated, use Wellbutrin (see chapter 3); it augments energy and concentration, and decreases pain.

Effexor is tolerated by most FMS sufferers in my practice, but one must start with the low dose in order to induce tolerance in the body for the higher doses. You should not begin at a 150-milligram dose. In fact, as one builds the dose, one may see a lessening of side effects. We ask our patients to take this drug immediately after breakfast to decrease the insomnia side effect. Occasionally, one might see elevated blood pressure, so B/P readings should be followed at home and certainly at the office. However, this side effect may be a blessing since many FMS and CFS patients suffer from hypotension. An increase or decrease in weight and sexual dysfunction may occur. When these side effects occur, I add Wellbutrin to augment the effectiveness of this medicine, to decrease the weight gain and to improve sexual dysfunction. When Effexor is not tolerated at all, I prescribe Wellbutrin in its place. (See chapter 3 for details on Wellbutrin.)

Daytime Pain Relief

Specific daytime pain relief can be achieved with muscle relaxants, benzodiazepines and narcotics. Flexeril is the best choice in my experience, and it is very effective. It is nondrowsy generally and can be used in the daytime or at night as an adjunct for sleep. It can also be used three to four times a day at the 10-milligram dose. Of course, it works in FMS because of its central—not its peripheral—actions. It is nonaddictive.

Narcotics

Narcotics are controversial in their use with FMS. Personally, I try to avoid narcotics, but I do use Ultram, since it is nonaddicting. Although it is a mild analgesic, it is chemically related to Effexor and therefore has several advantages. Its optimum pain relief, however, may take several weeks.

Benzodiazepines

The one benzodiazepine that is most recommended by the experts is Klonopin because of its superior effect on sleep architecture.

It is an antiepileptic, atypical benzodiazepine that has mild CNS antipain effects and anti-NMDA activity.[16] It has a relatively short half-life and is clearly superior to other benzodiazepines for sleep. This medicine also helps restless leg syndrome, if that is a problem. Certainly, if the price of the medicines is a problem, Klonopin can be chosen in lieu of the GABA agents Ambien or Sonata. If Klonopin is used during the day for fatigue or pain, it is more advantageous than Xanax or Ativan, since the addictive potential is less. Though the benzodiazepines are not characterized as pain relievers, they do relieve pain and fatigue in FMS and CFS, and it is probably because of their down-regulation of the NMDA receptors. It is believed that they relieve neurotoxicity of FMS and CFS.

Sleep Medications

The nonaddicting GABA agents such as zolpidem, Ambien, zaleplon and Sonata appear to have the least adverse effect on sleep architecture and are short acting. Ambien seems to be the most effective in FMS. The brain chemical GABA is very important in the initiation and maintenance of sleep. These agents virtually never cause hangover, even when taken as little as two hours before wake time. I especially choose these agents if an adjunct to a TCA or Zanaflex is needed. They can be used in two ways:

1. To help sleep onset
2. To continue the sleep cycle in the middle of the night

Melatonin at three to six milligrams is a very helpful sleep aid in some patients. This natural approach is safe and also has additional antioxidant protection. It also down-regulates NMDA receptor hyperactivity—one of the culprits of CFS and FMS—and helps protect the hippocampus, which is atrophied in FMS. I also recommend DHEA and natural progesterone in some cases because of their positive effect on dopamine levels.

MY MOST SUCCESSFUL TREATMENTS

Pharmacological	Natural	Procedures
Effexor XR	Melatonin	Vaccine neu-
Elavil or other TCA	Omega-3 EFAs	tralization
Wellbutrin	DHEA	Allergy immu-
Klonopin, Ambien	Antioxidants	notherapy
or Sonata	Magnesium/	(Only if signifi-
Zanaflex	Zinc	cant allergy
Flexeril	Natural Proges-	symptoms exist.
Neurontin	terone	See chapter 3.)
Benzodiazepines	Glutathione	
Narcotics (carefully)		
Pindolol		
Pindolol		

CONCLUSION

Obviously, treating patients with fibromyalgia requires much more than just diagnosing the condition and prescribing medication. Since FMS has such a wide variety of potential triggers, it's essential to listen carefully to each patient and get to know the physical and mental stresses that have been occurring in his or her life. Only then can you provide the individualized treatment and level of care that the patient needs. Taking the time to discuss all symptoms and possible causes—all concerns about what is happening to their body—and then providing hope for improvement can be just as therapeutic as drug treatment. Each of these patients has put their trust in you to be their lifeline to a healthier future.

FURTHER READING

Mitchell, S. M., et al. "Sleep in Chronic Pain: Problems and Treatments." *International Review of Psychiatry,* vol. 12 (2000), pp. 115-121.

Spitzer, Manfred. *The Mind Within the Net: Models of Learning, Thinking and Acting.* Cambridge, MA: The MIT Press, 1999, pp. 137-138.

Starz, Terrance. *Fibroymyalgia Network: Report of 2002 ACA Meeting,* 60th ed. (2003), pp. 3-4.

Ward, Dean. "Mitochondrial Dysfunction, Nutrition and Aging." *Vitamin Research News,* vol. 16, no. 10 (October 2002), pp. 1-14.

Watkins, L. A., and S. F. Maier. *Physical Revelation,* vol. 82, no. 4 (2002), pp. 981-1011.

CHAPTER 5

HIDDEN HYPOTHYROIDISM

Hypothyroidism is a condition in which the thyroid gland becomes underactive. Thyroid hormones (T4 and T3) are involved in producing energy and governing metabolism, so a deficiency can cause fatigue. Common symptoms include unexplained weight gain, muscle weakness, low-body temperature, inability to tolerate cold, hair loss and dry skin. The severity of the symptoms depends on the degree of hormone deficiency. Hidden hypothyroidism is simply hypothyroidism that is severe enough to cause troublesome symptoms but too mild to be diagnosed by a blood test. (In overt hypothyroidism, blood test results show the T4 and T3 levels to be low, with elevated TSH. Therefore, it is

One can have true hypothyroidism with a seemingly normal thyroid profile on a blood test. This disease is commonly missed yet easily treatable.

much simpler to diagnose.) This condition also is sometimes called subclinical hypothyroidism, decreased thyroid reserve and early thyroid failure.

Hidden hypothyroidism is arguably the most common cause of chronic fatigue in America and one of the least diagnosed. Most studies agree that the prevalence of the condition is probably between 5 and 10 percent of the general population. The key to diagnosis is to recognize that one can have true hypothyroidism with a seemingly normal thyroid profile on a blood test. This disease is commonly missed yet easily treatable. I believe the reason it is not diagnosed is because the clinician places more credibility on a lab test than on the patient and his or her history. The common practice of physicians diagnosing hypothyroidism based solely upon the thyroid lab test needs to stop.

SYMPTOMS

In addition to fatigue, I look for the four Cs that describe the hypothyroid patient:

1. Coldness
2. Constipation
3. Cramps (muscle)
4. Concentration problems

Along with hair loss and weight gain, these are the most common complaints of hypothyroidism. Some clinicians rely heavily on low body temperature, but this symptom on its own is unreliable, because there are many variables that control body temperature.

The following story depicts a 50-year-old hypothyroid female patient:

Several years ago, I began noticing memory loss, weight gain, hair loss, cold intolerance, dry skin and a feeling of total exhaustion. At the time, I was teaching an aerobics class. It became very embarrassing standing up in front of the class and being unable to remember the routines. The weight gain was obvious to everyone, and I just cried because I looked terrible even though I had good eating habits and was exercising. Eventually, I was so tired that I couldn't teach the class any more. Soon depression came.

I went to a doctor and blood work was done. He told me there was nothing wrong with me. He said hair loss was hereditary, weight gain was middle-age spread, memory loss was age-related, and he dismissed me as just "another complaining woman." My symptoms continued to get worse. I finally heard of Dr. Forester and made an appointment. He listened to my symptoms, and even before blood work was done, he told me I probably had a low thyroid condition. The results of my lab test said my thyroid was in normal range, but a small dose of Synthroid was prescribed and increased very slowly. I began feeling much better, and the depression eventually resolved.

After about 10 years, the Synthroid was no longer working and he changed me to Armor thyroid. Once again, my quality of life greatly improved. I've had my ups and downs with hypothyroidism, but with Armor thyroid and my doctor's help, I have overcome so many obstacles. I also have learned how to decrease my stress level and have taken aggressive control of my life. If I can feel better, I can help others. I thank God every day for my life, my health and my doctor.

Hypothyroid Symptom Checklist

____ I feel sluggish and tired a lot.

____ I feel down and depressed.

____ I'm gaining weight, even though I'm eating less.

____ I'm sleeping more than usual.

____ I'm often constipated.

____ I have some difficulty with concentration and memory.

____ I'm less interested in sex than usual.

____ My hair feels dry and brittle.

____ I haven't had a period for several months.

____ My periods have been irregular with lighter bleeding.

____ My voice sounds deeper and huskier than normal.

____ I feel stiff when I get out of bed in the morning.

____ My skin is dry and scaly.

____ I feel cold, even when others around me are comfortable.

____ My nails are brittle and grow in more slowly than usual.

____ I'm getting puffy around my eyes.

____ I have hair loss.

____ I have leg cramps.

Because symptoms such as fatigue, forgetfulness and weight gain can easily be attributed to other causes and because they tend to come on gradually, hypothyroidism is often misdiagnosed. A simple blood test can quickly confirm overt hypothyroidism. However, hidden hypothyroidism is more difficult to diagnose. Hormone levels are irregular enough to cause a patient to feel unwell, but they do not show up as abnormal in a blood test. Some patients continually test in the low-normal range of thyroid function and, therefore, do not receive treatment, even though they actually are suffering from this disease.

A case in point concerns a 58-year-old woman who was referred to me by a friend who found out about my treatment of migraines. The patient had been to some major headache clinics in America as well as some medical schools and, for approximately 20 years, had suffered from recurring and untreatable migraines. However, when she came to my office, her history revealed that she also was chronically fatigued and had many of the symptoms listed on the questionnaire for thyroid disease. I then obtained a thyroid profile and a sedimentation rate. I was so convinced that her symptoms were low thyroid that I told her I anticipated this diagnosis. Though her profile was normal, I started her on low doses of Synthroid, increasing to a level where she felt healthy again. Her husband said, "After 20 years, I finally got my wife back." Not only were her migraines resolved, but her fatigue and quality of life also were greatly improved.

Cause

This disease is basically a result of an autoimmune process in which the thyroid gland itself is attacked by the body. The body mistakenly develops antibodies that attack the thyroid gland, which causes inflammation and ultimately destruction of the thyroid tissue. Hidden hypothyroidism should be easily diagnosable; but, sadly, the parameters for diagnosis are inaccurate at best.

I remind my patients who have a borderline low thyroid or hidden hypothyroidism that physicians years ago depended upon the patient's history and physical exam rather than fancy tests to diagnose this condition and, therefore, they were probably more accurate in diagnosing hypothyroidism. Blood tests are valuable, but they are never to be used in lieu of how a patient feels and the symptoms that he or she describes to the physician.

This is one of the great mistakes of medicine in the twenty-first century. Data seem to have more credibility than the patient's symptoms for some physicians. Keep looking until you find a family practice or primary-care physician who will listen to you.

TREATMENT

The release of the thyroid hormone thyroxin (T4) is regulated by a higher brain function. When the brain senses low thyroid hormone in the bloodstream, the thyroid-releasing factor in the hypothalamus stimulates the pituitary to release thyroid-stimulating hormone (TSH) to cause the thyroid gland to manu-facture and release T4. After T4 is released into the bloodstream, it is converted by various organs of the body into tri-iodothyronine (T3), which is more active in regulating metabolism. T3 causes an increase in energy and performs other important functions. In the brain, thyroxine is a natural antidepressant.

The drug of choice for treating hypothyroidism is levothy-roxine (brand names Levoxyl and Synthroid). This drug contains a synthetic copy of the hormone T4, which is then converted by the body to T3. There is more to hypothyroidism than just a low release of T4. Not only is the thyroid gland unable to produce adequate amounts of thyroid, but the release of the hormones themselves induces an inflammatory response that can also cause an individual to feel ill. Therefore, when you take replace-ment thyroid medication, you not only gain supplementation for that part which the gland cannot release, but you also attain rest of the thyroid gland. This resting of the thyroid gland caus-es it to release a lower level of hormones, thereby decreasing the inflammatory response to that hormone. These are two impor-tant reasons why replacement medication helps the individual.

Thyroid medicine should be taken upon waking up in the morning—even before breakfast. This is very important because of the nature of the function of T4. If for some reason you do not respond to one type of thyroid medication, it is appropriate to change to another kind. When a person actually gains weight on Synthroid or a Synthroid-type product, it may mean that he or she is getting too much T4. In this case, it is advisable to switch to another kind of thyroid that includes T3 in its formula, which induces a natural weight loss. One also can take a lower dose of Synthroid and add Cytomel—T3—to that dose. Please note that it is unacceptable and unhealthy to use thyroid medicines for weight loss when one is not low thyroid.

EUTHYROID SICK SYNDROME

Another thyroid dysfunction that causes fatigue is called the euthyroid sick syndrome. In his textbook *Endocrine Secrets*, Dr. Michael McDermot, professor of medicine, division of endocrinology, at the University of Colorado School of Medicine, describes this syndrome. It occurs when a nonthyroidal illness such as infection, heart attack, trauma, cancer or other inflammatory condition causes an irregularity of thyroid levels. The thyroid gland itself is not diseased or inflamed. Other factors in the body of the ill person are causing the imbalance of thyroid hormones. Usually, these patients have a low T3 level because T4 is not being converted to T3 due to the presence of inflammatory cytokines. The blood test results are characterized by normal TSH and normal T4 but low T3. [1] This syndrome is not well known in the medical community, but it is real and has been reported in various publications, including the journal *Thyroid*. [2]

Another cause of this syndrome could possibly be the use of synthetic hormones such as women's birth control pills. All synthetic hormones cause an antibody response, which includes cytokine-based inflammation. This could potentially have an effect on the thyroid gland, which may explain the number of cases of euthyroid sick syndrome that I see in women. Indeed, this could become a major health problem in Western medicine. I have discovered that many CFS and FMS patients have euthyroid sick syndrome. The addition of lower doses of thyroid medication makes a big difference in their quality of life.

CONCLUSION

1. You may have low thyroid and still have what appears to be a normal blood test.
2. Your history and how you feel are vital in determining if you have low thyroid.
3. It is *okay* to start thyroid hormone replacement at low doses and increase carefully until one feels normal.
4. Hypothyroidism is one of many illnesses that can cause you to feel tired.
5. Find a doctor who will listen to you, and stay with him or her.

TO THE PHYSICIAN

HIDDEN HYPOTHYROIDISM

Epidemiology   Increasingly common

Key symptoms and history   1. Slow onset
2. Chronic fatigue
3. Coldness

Continued on next page

Continued from previous page

	4. Hair loss
	5. Weight gain or difficulty losing weight
Diagnosis	Fairly simple if patient's history rather than lab test is relied on
Treatment approach	1. Simple
	2. Side effects uncommon
Prognosis	1. Excellent if recognized
	2. Virtually 100% curable

In 1994, I gave a short talk at the American Academy of Otolaryngic Allergy Symposium in New Orleans. I had been given authority by the society's executive committee to help recruit primary-care doctors to our allergy society. At the refreshment break, I began conversing with Dr. Allen McDaniel, one of the symposium lecturers and a recipient of a number of research grants. He also teaches part-time at a local ear, nose and throat residency program.

Dr. McDaniel stated that he had just completed a research project on occult hypothyroidism. He discovered that patients who had symptoms of low thyroid but had normal lab tests—including antithyroid antibodies—were found to be truly low thyroid. He proved this by doing needle biopsies of their thyroid glands, and subsequent pathology reports proved that these patients had sick glands. This was astonishing to me since I had never heard of any such research. I had patients with classic hypothyroid symptoms, even though all tests appeared normal. Could it be that I was missing their true diagnosis?

I decided to use this approach with my patients who exhibited coldness, weight gain, hair loss and fatigue; and to my amazement, it worked! Approximately 90 to 95 percent of these fatigue patients who had low thyroid systems showed dramatic improvement in their quality of life after treatment. Since then, I have discovered literally hundreds of patients with what I now term hidden hypothyroidism.

Several authorities have documented the necessity to lower the normal range for TSH, or thyroid-stimulating hormone, in blood tests. The original guidelines for TSH were set at seven. Later that was reduced to five. Now it is four and a half. But fairly recently, Dr. L. M. Demers of the National Academy of Clinical Biochemistries, stated:

> In the future, it is likely that the upper of the serum TSH euthyroid reference range will be reduced to 2.5 because less than 95% of rigorously screened normal euthyroid volunteers have serum TSH values between 0.4 and 2.5.[3]

Another thyroid specialist, Dr. Richard Shames, coauthor of the book *Thyroid Power*, states that physicians ignore the advice that is given in the *Physician's Desk Reference*. The drug company Knoll, which makes Synthroid, advises that physicians should not depend solely on a particular blood test (TSH, T3 and T4) to diagnose or manage low thyroid. One should use the patient's history and physical exam, as well as the laboratory data, to render this diagnosis. Dr. Shames strongly asserts that no one test or series of tests should be utilized by health-care professionals to rule out hypothyroidism.[4]

If TSH—which has been relied on for years—is not sensitive enough to detect all thyroid disease, then which test is? Dr. Ridha Arem, chair of Endocrinology at Baylor, states that the suppression test is the most accurate test to determine if one has low thyroid.[5] However, this test is generally done at medical schools and is very expensive. Dr. J. C. Lowe agrees that a TSH may not be sufficient to diagnose hypothyroidism. Normal lab results do not rule it out. In addition, he strongly asserts that most FMS patients have hypothyroidism.[6] I have found this to be true in my practice. Most of my FMS patients fit the euthyroid sick syndrome profile.

DIAGNOSIS

In diagnosing hypothyroidism, I first order a thyroid profile and usually a sed. rate at the same time. Sed. rate is a measure of inflammation—if the thyroid is under attack, the ESR will be somewhat elevated. Sometimes we will proceed to antithyroid antibody testing, which actually picks up the immune factors that are attacking the gland. The thyroid peroxidase antibody (TPO) test can be helpful in diagnosis as well.

If the patient does have hidden hypothyroidism, there will usually be a hint of low T4 or borderline T4 or T3, but the patient's history will always correlate with these abnormal findings. The chairman of the medicine department at Medical College of Georgia in Augusta (where I trained) once said, "If you listen to the patient long enough, he will tell you what's wrong with him." Today, many of us are *not* listening to patients. Rather, we are relying on tests. It is in the patient's history that one will usually diagnose hypothyroidism. I have my patients fill out a

Many doctors are not listening to patients. Rather, they are relying on tests. It is in the patient's history that doctors will usually diagnose hypothyroidism.

questionnaire that includes the hypothyroid symptom check-list (see earlier in this chapter). If this questionnaire strongly suggests thyroid disease, and a thyroid profile is borderline, I usually will start Synthroid at low doses and increase the dose to about 100 micrograms. Then I will retest the patient after the 100-microgram dose has been taken for approximately three weeks—to see where their profile is and how they feel. I will modify doses up or down accordingly. As the patient slowly increases his or her doses in 50-microgram increments, he or she may start to feel high or jittery. I then tell the patient either to go back to the previous dose or to stop the Synthroid. In less than 5 percent of my patients have I seen this happen. In spite of reports to the contrary, there are a growing number of physicians, including myself, who believe that a TSH level as low as .1 is safe, as long as the patient feels well and his or her vital signs and physical exam are normal.[7]

CASE STUDY

A 42-year-old male schoolteacher came to the clinic and stated that he had been fatigued and had swelling in his extremities for approximately five to seven years. He was on 60 to 80 milligrams of Prozac a day and 120 milligrams of Lasix for his extremity edema. Still, the patient felt very tired and depressed and had a poor quality of life. His thyroid profile, including T3, T4 and TSH, was basically within normal limits; but his T3 was slightly low, and his sedimentation rate was slightly elevated. His questionnaire was strongly positive for thyroid disease, so I started him on increasing doses of Synthroid. To his utter amazement, he began feeling like his old self again, and his Lasix was eventually discontinued. His Prozac dosage was lowered to 20 milligrams a day instead of 60 milligrams a day. He was indeed very grateful, especially because he was a single father raising five children and needed all the energy and emotional stamina he could muster.

TREATMENT

What kind of thyroid medication should one use? Probably the most often used thyroid medication in the United States is Synthroid. It is a synthetic molecule that is made up of T4. T4 then is converted to T3 by enzymatic systems in the body. The advantage of Synthroid is that the body is not barraged by powerful T3, as in some drugs, but converts T4 to T3 as the need arises. T3 supplementation alone can be overly activating and, in some people, can cause cardiac arrhythmias. But in some cases, adding T3 as part of a medication may be necessary, since some patients poorly convert T4 to T3.

Another form of thyroid medication is armor thyroid, which is made from swine but is considered natural and is used by older primary-care physicians as well as many doctors who practice natural medicine. It is composed of approximately 95 percent T4 and 5 percent T3. The T3 is released quickly and gives a spurt of energy, and the T4 is converted as described above.

Levoxyl, Levothroid and Unithroid are three other T4-type medications that are used by physicians and clinicians to treat the disease. They too are effective.

Cytomel, a synthetic T3, is available and is used by thyroid specialists to augment the T4-type medications and to modify how patients feel. There also are some physicians who use Cytomel for depressive and low-energy symptoms in some patients. This form of the hormone is rather short-acting but very effective.

There are some physicians who criticize my approach, stating that it is treating patients blindly with only anecdotal evidence. My response is that I treat the patient, not a lab test. It is simple to diagnose thyroid disease when the TSH is obviously abnormal. It takes clinical skill and the ability to simply listen to patients to diagnose accurately subclinical disease. Let me hasten to add that if evidenced by lab data or clinical symptoms the patient becomes hyperthyroid, I reduce dosage or stop the medicine.

CHAPTER 6

YEAST OVERGROWTH SYNDROME

Candidiasis

Perhaps the most underdiagnosed and least understood of all the fatigue syndromes is the candida overgrowth hypersensitivity syndrome (COS), or yeast overgrowth syndrome. The reality of this syndrome was at first questioned by many clinicians, but it has recently gained support by a number of authorities who teach at such medical schools as Harvard, Tulane and the University of Southern California. It also has been accepted as fact by several national scientific societies, and doctors across the nation who treat this condition are growing in number. I personally have diagnosed and treated hundreds of patients (including myself) with this condition since 1991.

Candida albicans is a common yeast that lives in the mouth, digestive tract, genital tract and skin. It ordinarily does no harm because a healthy body can keep it under control. Certain friend-ly, or probiotic, bacteria limit the growth of yeast colonies. If these friendly bacteria are weak and low in number, candida can develop into an invasive form and penetrate mucus membranes throughout the body. This candida overgrowth, or candidiasis, can cause various problems, depending on whether the over-growth is localized or systemic (affecting the whole body). For instance, a candida infection in the mouth is called thrush. Localized candida also can infect the female genital tract, caus-ing a discharge and itching and burning.

SYMPTOMS

Systemic candidiasis, or yeast overgrowth syndrome, causes symptoms that include fatigue, allergic reactions, heartburn, constipation, diarrhea, colitis, rectal itching, bloating and cramps, kidney and bladder infections, muscle and joint pain, sore throat, cough and nasal congestion, numbness or tingling of the extremities and fungal infections of the nails. Weakness, hyperactivity, blood-sugar regulation problems, headaches, memory problems and depression also have been attributed to yeast overgrowth.

The primary symptom of this syndrome is fatigue—some-times severe—in virtually every patient with the illness. The fatigue, however, may be attributed to another condition such as depression, anxiety, CFS, fibromyalgia, irritable bowel syn-drome, or the like. The gastrointestinal tract is a major target of yeast overgrowth, and a sufferer of this condition usually experi-ences dull abdominal aching, indigestion, diarrhea or loose stools, or constipation, which may mimic irritable bowel syn-drome. Decreased libido and lowered sexual performance are very common. The mental aspects are very disconcerting. Poor concentration, memory loss and brain fog are almost always associated with the condition; sometimes anxiety and panic are associated with it as well.[1]

Yeast overgrowth can cause the following problems:

- Chronic fatigue
- Muscle aches
- Joint pains
- Impaired memory
- Lack of the ability to concentrate
- Digestive disorders
- Confusion
- Sleep disturbance
- Weakness
- Irritability
- Allergic reactions
- Headaches
- Diarrhea
- Rectal itching
- Sore throat, cough and nasal congestion

BACKGROUND

In spite of the information and evidence that exists, there remains a certain amount of ignorance and disbelief about the existence of candidiasis. However, in the prestigious infectious disease textbook *Principles and Practice of Infectious Disease,* the factual history is clear:

The most interesting period in the history of Candida infections began in the 1940s when the widespread use of antibiotics was introduced. Since then, previously undocumented manifestations of Candida infections have occurred, and the incidence of practically all forms of

Candida infections has risen abruptly. Candida species are now the fourth most common organisms recovered from blood of hospitalized patients in the United States.[2]

The use of broad-spectrum antibiotics suppresses bacterial species in the colon and GI tract and, therefore, allows candida to proliferate. In particular, certain antibiotics such as sulfonamides, tetracycline, doxycycline and aminoglycosides decrease the ability of the white blood cells to kill the candida. This information is clearly stated in a major, traditional infectious disease textbook. Therefore, there is clear historical evidence that the dramatic increase in candidal infections is directly related to the widespread use of antibiotics. As a physician and a pharmacologist, I am thankful for the discovery and widespread availability of antibiotics. But with the good comes the bad—with a marvelous advancement in the treatment of infectious disease, complications of such treatments are obvious. As I learned on the first day of my master's degree training in pharmacology, the first law of pharmacology is "No drug has a single effect."

There is clear historical evidence that the dramatic increase in candidal infections is directly related to the widespread use of antibiotics.

Just what is the nature of the yeast organism named *Candida albicans*, and how does it cause fatigue and other debilitating symptoms? Let's take a look.

EARLY HISTORY

It was 1953 and the use of antibiotics had been spreading for over a decade. Already, complications of antibiotic use, such as anaphylaxis and skin rashes, had been acknowledged and described in medical literature. One such complication, however, had not been recognized and, in large part, remains unrecognized today. In an Alabama hospital lay a very sick man who had not responded to therapy for approximately four months; his diagnosis was thereby inconclusive. A physician named Orian Truss made a simple observation after questioning the man as to when his condition began. The patient stated that after he had taken antibiotics for an injured finger, he developed diarrhea and other worsening symptoms. Dr. Truss was aware that candida was an opportunistic organism and thrived in immuno-compromised individuals; therefore, he surmised that candida overgrowth was actually the cause of this patient's condition. To put this theory to the test, he gave the patient a medicine called Lugol's solution (potassium iodide), and within a matter of days the patient recovered and was restored to his normal state of health. Dr. Truss tried similar therapy for a female patient who had been on antibiotics and complained of headaches, severe depression and vaginal symptoms; and her problems resolved. He even saw a dramatic response in a woman who was diagnosed as schizophrenic and had undergone multiple drug therapies and shock treatments. She was restored to normal mental health and required no further psychiatric intervention after candidal treatment was given. In this particular patient, Dr. Truss used a candida neutralization technique for her allergies. Because of the success of this procedure along with a combination of anti-fungal medications and a low-sugar diet, he had discovered a treatment for this "new" illness. Upon confirmation of his findings by other physicians—similarly impressed at the incredible improvement in their patients—he presented his observations in a medical symposium in 1977. By 1981, he published what some believe is a landmark paper entitled "The Role of *Candida albicans* in Human Illness." His book *The Missing Diagnosis* soon followed.

Further research revealed that certain toxins produced by

the presence of candida in the gut seemed to explain some of the systemic symptoms—including fatigue—observed in patients suffering from candida overgrowth syndrome. It became apparent that the consumption of simple sugars was a strong risk factor in the development of the illness. In fact, Dr. Truss discovered that most patients actually craved sugar. Could it be that a fermentation process was occurring in the gut, the same way yeast causes dough to rise? Additionally, was there an immune response to fermentation chemicals or to the candida itself, which could explain the illness? I will answer these questions later, but let's continue the story.

As the word spread among physicians and incredible results were seen in their fatigued patients, a pediatrician and allergist named Dr. William Crook from Jackson, Tennessee, became especially interested in the subject. He began writing a series of books and entitled the first one *The Yeast Connection.*[3] The title of that book is a common term used for COS today. Additionally, his efforts to disseminate the information are unparalleled over the last two decades; and, in my opinion, he is one of the world's foremost authorities on the subject.

Instead of relying on anecdotal information alone, Dr. Crook has consistently asked the traditional community to investigate the subject of candidal infections and to perform studies that would give light to what he called the yeast connection. Because of his courage and persistence and the establishment of a nonprofit organization named the International Health Foundation, thousands of suffering patients who were in despair have been helped.

PERSONAL EXPERIENCE

When I first heard of the yeast overgrowth syndrome in 1988, I was very skeptical, like many physicians. The patient who brought a copy of *The Yeast Connection* to me was convinced that what the author had to say was true, while I was equally convinced it was another scam. In 1991, I became interested in the field of allergy and furthered my education through seminars sponsored by the Pan American Allergy Society and continuing education courses offered by the American Academy of Otolaryngic Allergy. As I listened to lectures from physicians who were outstanding in the field of allergy and immunology, I found that this yeast syndrome was, indeed, a believable entity. Some of the lecturers were teaching at residency programs in various medical schools.

I carried the simple techniques learned at these seminars back to my clinic in Pineville, Louisiana, and found that a number of patients with fatigue had a yeast problem. By the fall of 1996, I found myself suffering from worsening fatigue and myalgias over the course of several months. Routine lab tests and X rays were normal. To me, it was a complete enigma. The achiness, fatigue and brain fog would not respond to Advil, Naprosyn or Tylenol. I was puzzled almost to the point of despair and began to make plans to have an extensive diagnostic workup at Ochsner Clinic Foundation in New Orleans. At the suggestion of Cheryl, my wife and soul mate in the Lord, I treated myself with the antifungal medication Diflucan, and the symptoms resolved. After such dramatic improvement, it was obvious I did not need the million-dollar diagnostic workup. I only needed a 25-dollar prescription of antifungal medication, acidophilus and an appropriate diet.

I can say with confidence that the scientific data, treatment of my patients and my own personal experience prove that the candida overgrowth syndrome is valid. One must remember that not everyone with fatigue has a yeast problem; yet, it is certainly one of the easiest of the syndromes to treat, and it is gratifying to see patients improve after suffering for months or years.

One such patient was a registered nurse who heard about my successful approach to chronic fatigue syndrome. Although prescribed an antidepressant by her internist, she continued to experience fatigue, brain fog and aching. The easy clue of COS in her history was that the symptoms began after intense treatment of intravenous antibiotics approximately two years previously. Within two to three days after starting antifungal medication, she made a startling improvement. On follow-up, she was given a low-sugar diet and, as far as I know, she continues in remission.

YEAST GROWTH

Yeasts are considered true fungi and, under the microscope, they look like spaghetti and meatballs. They divide by budding or direct division. Yeasts are found in nature on leaves and flowers and in soil and salt water. These organisms are specifically known to ferment simple sugars, and certain kinds are used in producing alcoholic beverages such as beer and wine, or in baking bread. In the latter, the fermentation of baker's yeast gives off carbon dioxide and alcohol. The gas, carbon dioxide, is trapped in tiny bubbles and causes the dough to expand and rise.

Yeasts are considered true fungi and they divide by budding or direct division.

It is apparent that the cause of the multiple symptoms of COS, which Walter Last calls the antibiotic syndrome, is ascribed to an apparent overgrowth of yeast in the intestinal tract. The GI tract is warm and moist, and the pH balance of the large intestine is perfect for candida to grow and thrive. Deterring the rapid multiplication of candida is a function of the millions of friendly bacteria that normally exist in this environment. Yeast and bacteria are both essential in the body, and they are an example of a precisely balanced symbiotic relationship. Since this balance is critical, one can easily understand that when antibiotics kill off friendly bacteria, candida and other types of microbiologic agents are allowed to grow.

The four pathogenic mechanisms that have been postulated to explain the symptoms of candida overgrowth are the following:

1. **An Immunologic or Allergic Reaction.** The body has an incredibly complex protective system, which is absolutely necessary for health. This immune system will react to invaders in an attempt to eradicate the threat of infection. Many times, the immune system overreacts, such as in an allergic response. Many infections cause the body to release cytokines, prostaglandins and other immune factors, which assist in the killing of antigens. This cytokine production actually plays a major role in the symptoms of the disease. For example, the common cold is caused by a virus that infects only the nose and the upper respiratory tract; but it affects several systems of the body, causing low-grade fevers, aching, chills and general malaise (fatigue). These symptoms are caused by the immune response mentioned earlier. The virus itself only induces the symptoms related to the nose. The same is true with the influenza virus, which only affects the lungs. The fever, chills and weakness are symptoms caused by the immune system itself. In the same way, there is good evidence that the hypersensitive immune response to the presence of fast-multiplying yeast organisms causes the multiple symptoms of the candida syndrome.

2. **Toxic Waste Products.** It has been proven that the candida organism can release or produce up to 79 different

toxins, which can, in turn, be absorbed by the intestines into the body.[4] One such chemical is D-arabitol. This sugar metabolite has been shown to be toxic to the brain and nervous system. But perhaps the major toxin that produces damage in the body is the candidal waste product, acetaldehyde.[5] Aldehyde is thought to be responsible for many of the health problems associated with alcoholism, including muscle damage to the heart. It also is poisonous to the brain, spinal cord, joints and muscles, producing irritation and pain. Fatigue is a major result of acetaldehyde intoxication, and Dr. Orian Truss, the discoverer of the yeast syndrome, considers much of the damage done by candida to be caused by this chemical. As long as the candida organisms remain in small numbers in the gut, these toxic effects are not an issue at all. But when their numbers are allowed to increase dramatically, *watch out*, for you may end up feeling worse than drunk. Some researchers and clinicians feel that some of the toxins released induce certain receptors in the brain to turn on an intense desire for sugars. As one craves and consumes these sugars, the food supply of the candida is increased and allows for the yeast overgrowth cycle to continue.

3. **Allergic Food Reaction.** There are two basic kinds of food allergies: fixed and cyclic. A fixed food allergy is one in which the body's immune system is considered to be permanently hypersensitive to a certain food. Once a person has come in contact with a certain offending food, that person's body becomes sensitized. A second dose of that food produces a significant reaction termed "anaphylaxis." This reaction can be life threatening because it causes air hunger, asthma and

possibly shock and hypotension. The treatment is an immediate injection of epinephrine followed by antihistamines and steroids. The only way to prevent this significant reaction is to avoid the food; there are no allergy shots that are safe and effective to prevent this reaction from taking place.

However, the second type of food allergy, cyclic, is much more subtle and usually not serious. It involves other types of immune factors that may not be life threatening but can make a sufferer feel ill. The person may experience symptoms immediately or hours after the food has been consumed and metabolized. Runny nose, headache, muscle aches, joint pains, skin rashes and itching are common reactions. This type of food allergy is difficult to identify, because the allergic response may occur hours after the food is eaten. The treatment for this cyclic type of food allergy is simply to discontinue a suspect food for several months, allowing the body's immune system to calm down. Then the person is usually able to eat the particular food every three to four days without side effects. However, if the food is eaten daily or several times a day, then the original symptoms may recur. It is felt by many clinicians that the presence of large amounts of intestinal yeast produces this sensitivity to certain foods.

4. **Leaky Gut.** The candidal syndrome can cause damage to the normal lining of the intestines. This damage allows larger molecules of food to be absorbed, producing what some clinicians have called a leaky gut. Since the body is not used to these larger molecules, it sets up an immune, allergic reaction to the apparent foreign invader. The reaction can be felt in any system

of the body, depending upon the nature of the macro-molecule and the particular chemistry and immunity of the individual. This leaky gut syndrome is more closely related to the cyclic food allergy than it is to the fixed food allergy. If the intestines are rid of the overabundance of candida organisms, the body then will repair the damage to the gut, and the food allergies will eventually disappear.

CAUSES

There are three main factors that predispose a person to candida overgrowth:

1. **Impaired immune function.** This can be temporary—the result of chemotherapy or steroid treatment—or it can be long-term—as in HIV disease and certain cancers.
2. **Destruction of friendly bacteria.** Friendly bacteria are destroyed by antibiotic therapy primarily, but stress and the aging process can contribute to a decline as well.
3. **The presence of an abundance of sugar.** Sugar is a food source for yeast and encourages them to grow. People with diabetes are more prone to candida infections than most, but anyone whose diet consists of mostly sugary and yeast-based foods is susceptible.

Other factors that predispose a person to candida overgrowth include:

• Antibiotic usage greater than two to four weeks
• Childhood treatment for such things as ear infections

- The use of steroids or immunosuppressants
- The use of birth control pills or female hormones
- Intake and/or craving of sugars and simple carbohydrates
- A history of major surgery after which the fatigue began
- Multiple pregnancies

DIET TREATMENT

The COS diet has similarities to the diabetic or sugar buster's diet, which greatly limits sugar, junk foods and most white foods. White foods turn to sugar in your body and feed the candida organisms. Therefore, the following substitutions are recommended:

- Whole grain bread for white bread
- Brown rice for white rice
- Whole grain pasta for white pasta
- Sweet potato for white potato (or eat a white potato *and* its skin)

You also need to limit or completely discontinue sugary beverages and use either saccharin or the new sweetener, Splenda, for sugar substitutes, both of which research says are safe. I strongly believe that NutraSweet is detrimental to one's health and is a "poisonous" food additive. In your body, it may be metabolized to formaldehyde and/or methyl alcohol in quantities that produce physical effects such as migraine headaches, memory loss and, reportedly, elevated blood sugars in some diabetics. One patient, a pharmacist, told me that when she discontinued all NutraSweet, she was also able to stop her antidepressants. We have found Diet Rite Cola, which contains no caffeine and does contain Splenda, to be a very good cola substitute.

Both my wife and I were experiencing migraine headaches with the NutraSweet-containing colas but have noticed no apparent side effects from Diet Rite Cola.

Dr. William Crook in *The Yeast Connection and the Woman* states:

> Avoid yeasty foods and beverages, especially dried fruits, mushrooms, condiments, alcohol, juices except for freshly squeezed juices, leavened breads, bagels, pastries, pretzels, pizza and rolls. Two or three weeks after you improve, you can try a yeasty food and see if it bothers you. Diets aren't forever and, after a few weeks or months, you may be able to relax a bit; yet, until you show significant improvement, stick to your diet.[6]

Additionally, every day drink at least six to eight glasses of pure water to help flush toxins out of your system, and include olive oil in your diet. Yeasts do not feed well on fats, and olive oil is a beneficial fat, because it is monounsaturated. I strongly recommend lowering animal fat intake and eating more of the antioxidant-containing fresh vegetables and a moderate amount of fresh fruits, with the above exceptions. Plus, consume omega-3 fatty acids, which are beneficial and are obtained in natural flaxseed oil, ground flaxseeds and fish oil

Every day drink at least six to eight glasses of pure water to help flush toxins out of your system.

and in capsules. This essential fatty acid is great for lowering cholesterol, strengthening the immune system and improving nervous system function. Studies have shown that it also can help depression and bipolar illness. Vitamin/mineral supplements containing healthy doses of vitamins C and E are helpful in preventing and healing many illnesses. Several years ago it was taught in medical schools that vitamin supplements were not useful because the food we eat contains all of the nutrients that we need. It is interesting to note that today the majority of American physicians take supplements. Most cardiologists take vitamin E and C. Most ophthalmologists recommend folic acid and other vitamins. Psychiatrists are strongly recommending the omega-3 fatty acid supplements.

Finally, avoid alcoholic beverages, because they are fermented and contain yeasts, and the body breaks alcohol down into sugar. Do not eat foods with a high mold content, such as cheese, dried fruit, peanuts and melons. Eat several servings daily of foods that contain friendly bacteria, such as yogurt and acidophilus milk. You also may obtain healthy bacteria from probiotic supplements that contain acidophilus and bifidus. It is essential to restore the proper bacterial balance to control candida overgrowth.

Avoid consuming the following:

- All types of sugar (including fruit juice)
- Processed foods containing corn syrup and sugar
- White foods (white flour products, potatoes and rice)
- Foods containing yeast (read labels)
- Mold-containing foods (cheese, dried fruit, peanuts and melons)
- Alcohol

Do consume the following:

- Plain yogurt with live cultures (or acidophilus-fortified milk)
- Probiotic supplements
- Six to eight glasses of water per day

- Healthy oils (fish and olive oil)
- Whole grains (brown foods)
- Fresh vegetables

Medications that are effective in stopping yeast overgrowth include:

- Antifungal drugs (Flucanazole, Diflucan)
- Similar drugs (Sporanox, Nizoral and Lamisil)

For additional information, see the "To the Physician" section of this chapter.

CHILDREN AND ADOLESCENTS

Irritable Kids Syndrome

Yeast overgrowth syndrome can affect children as well as adults. Toddlers and young children will not generally complain of fatigue, but parents know something is wrong because of their actions. Fatigued kids do not sleep well. They cry easily, fret often and seem alternately agitated and lethargic. Many will have loose stools or diarrhea, and a virus may be blamed or another ear infection, though fever is not in the picture. Recurrent use of antibiotics and other therapies do not seem to help.

Symptoms may include:

- Irritability
- Crying spells
- Sleep difficulties
- Recurrent use of antibiotics
- Rashes
- Hyperactivity

The following is a typical case of a child suffering from irritable kids syndrome:

> A child has a true ear infection or sinusitis. The physician gives appropriate antibiotics, but many times follow-up antibiotics are needed. The child starts displaying symptoms as described above, and he or she is taken back to the physician who prescribes more antibiotics. Since the classic white tongue of thrush is not observed, the candidiasis syndrome is not suspected. Continual irritability and rashes or facial swelling may prompt the parents to consult an allergist or ear, nose and throat doctor. If the physician is astute and aware of the yeast overgrowth syndrome, then appropriate treatment can be given. I have seen a number of children dramatically improve who had symptoms as stated above, and I know there are literally thousands of toddlers and children who are suffering from the yeast overgrowth syndrome.

Diagnosis. An oral wet-prep or KOH taken from the child's mouth will usually reveal numerous yeast with spores. Under the microscope, it looks like spaghetti and meatballs.

This diagnosis is assured when one observes an incredible improvement after appropriate doses of Diflucan. Nystatin can also be given, but the improvement will be slower. In my experience, parents are usually amazed at the recovery of their child from the irritability and are usually very thankful to the physician.

Case Report. The parents of a 15-month-old child were on itinerant mission work in China. Grandparents were caring for the child and, knowing that I am an allergist, they brought the toddler to my office. The history was typical. After succumbing to numerous infections of the ears and sinuses and multiple treatments of antibiotics, the little one had exhibited the typical irritability as described above. He had been hospitalized approximately three months earlier with severe sinusitis. There was mild improvement in the interim, but the child again began to exhibit irritability, crying spells and insomnia. At the time, he was on a very strong broad-spectrum antibiotic. An oral swab revealed clumps of yeast and spores; therefore, liquid Diflucan was instituted while the antibiotics were discontinued. The next day, the grandparents called me and exclaimed that a miracle had occurred. The little one had slept well and awoke playful and happy. I prescribed a low sugar/starch diet and acidophilus such as Bacid capsules or Lactinex. I further emphasized to the grandparents that in the susceptible patient who is given antibiotics, Nystatin and acidophilus should be taken in order to prevent the same syndrome. When the parents arrived home from China, they were also amazed at the child's great improvement.

Irritable Adolescents Syndrome

A teen's presentation of symptoms is somewhat different than toddlers and children. They have symptoms more like adults, but from my experience, abdominal complaints usually predominate. Parents usually take their teenagers from specialist to specialist without a resolution of the problem.

Symptoms may include:

- Chronic fatigue
- Depression
- Possible hyperactivity or attention deficit
- Abdominal pain with diarrhea or constipation
- History of multiple antibiotic use
- Irritability

Case Report. A 14-year-old male, complaining chiefly of persistent abdominal pain and nausea, came to my office. He had a four-month history of progressing symptoms and, at this point, he was unable to attend school due to the severity of the problem. Several doctors had been consulted and extensive laboratory, radiological and endoscopic studies had been done with conclusions of only mild gastritis and chronic constipation; therefore, he was labeled as having irritable bowel syndrome. He was taking Prilosec, Phenergan, Levsin, Citrucel and being maintained on a high fiber diet; yet he continued to have abdominal cramping and nausea. Lack of energy, poor academic performance (by a previously straight-A student) and general apathy had been simply explained away as teenage behavioral problems. Because no conclusive diagnosis could be reached to match the weight of the problem, counseling was suggested; yet even there no conclusive psychological problem could be found, and the focus was to learn to deal with the chronic pain. My wife, a church friend of this young man's mother, knew of his problem and had been praying for him. She mentioned the yeast overgrowth syndrome and the success that we had with previous patients who had unexplainable abdominal pain. The young man came for an office visit and mentioned he had mononucleosis the previous year and was given multiple rounds of antibiotics and prednisone. I prescribed Diflucan, and after one treatment, he noted marked improvement in the abdominal cramping, and the nausea subsided. This regimen had to be repeated a few months later when cramping and inability to concentrate began again, but this round resulted in abatement of all symptoms and his ability to return to activities as normal.

Summary

In closing, the irritable kids and adolescents syndromes can be significant problems in children who have taken multiple antibiotics. Sometimes, the antibiotics are not even needed in the first place, since the original problem may be viral and not bacterial. But the physician may feel compelled to prescribe needless antibiotics due to pressure from the parents. When antibiotics are necessary, we suggest that acidophilus, yogurt or buttermilk be taken to prevent yeast overgrowth.

Here are important points to remember when dealing with irritable kids and adolescents syndromes:

1. Irritable kids and adolescents may have yeast overgrowth.
2. Yeasts liberate numerous toxins that produce the symptoms of these syndromes.
3. Diflucan is my drug of choice, but Nystatin can also be used.
4. Abdominal symptoms predominate in adolescents, while irritability and crying are usually seen in toddlers.
5. Medical authorities believe that there is an overuse of antibiotics in Western countries, and this overuse contributes to yeast overgrowth.

TO THE PHYSICIAN

YEAST OVERGROWTH SYNDROME

Epidemiology	Increasingly common, especially in children
Key symptoms and history	1. Rather abrupt after prolonged or frequent antibiotic use
	2. Chronic fatigue
	3. Brain fog

Continued on next page

Continued from previous page

	4. Insomnia, frequently accompanied by itching
	5. Sexual dysfunction
	6. Abdominal discomfort
Diagnosis	Simple if physician believes in syndrome; if not, virtually impossible
Treatment approach	1. Simple and straightforward
	2. Side effects uncommon
Prognosis	1. Excellent if recognized; poor if not
	2. Virtually 100% curable
	3. Relapses common

The following are the six most common symptoms of candida overgrowth syndrome:

1. Fatigue
2. Flu symptoms—achiness usually without fever
3. Mental problems, which include brain fog, depression and low concentration
4. Gastrointestinal problems, including dull aching pain in the abdomen with constipation and usually diarrhea or loose stools
5. Unexplained insomnia
6. Sexual side effects and/or vaginitis

The following are the most common predisposing factors:

- Prolonged antibiotic use—usually longer than 10 to 14 days (especially use of broad-spectrum agents)
- Use of birth control pills and hormones
- Inhalant and/or food allergies
- Chemical sensitivities
- Use of steroids or immunosuppressive agents
- Sugar cravings and ingestion of large amounts of simple sugars such as cookies, candy, junk foods, fruit juices and mold-containing foods
- Multiple pregnancies
- A history of major surgery (after which the fatigue began)

COS cause and effect overview:

- Numerous friendly bacterial species live in the colon. Long and/or strong antibiotics (or other causes) kill off native bacteria.
- Aggressive candida—normally low in number in the colon—overgrow (in susceptible patients).
- Steroids or estrogens may augment growth.
- Candida release toxins including alcohol and aldehydes.
- Proinflammatory cytokines react.
- The patient experiences fatigue, brain fog, abdominal discomfort and so on.
- The astute health-care provider recognizes the syndrome and prescribes anticandidal therapy (e.g., Diflucan).
- Low-sugar diet and probiotics, yogurt and/or butter-milk are recommended.
- The patient feels dramatically better as colon balance is renewed and the recommended diet is maintained.

CLINICAL/SCIENTIFIC ANALYSIS

If candida overgrowth syndrome is a real thing, if it is a significant cause of fatigue, then why isn't it well known and generally accepted by the medical community? First, I would say the wheels of medicine turn very slowly, especially if the discovery doesn't originate from a medical school or a pharmaceutical company. There are a number of examples in medical history, one of which has to do with allergies. It was many years before the science of allergy was even believed by general and primary-care physicians. After 20 to 40 years of giving allergy shots, allergists were vindicated when the IgE immunoglobulin was discovered. This biochemical is directly responsible for inhalant and many other allergic reactions.

Second, since candida is a normal inhabitant of the GI tract and in other mucous membranes of the body as well as the skin, and since there is no clear-cut invasion by these organisms into the tissues, it is difficult to make a case for a clinical syndrome or illness. One would think that stool cultures would reveal the presence of infections; and, in fact, gram stains do reveal yeast in increased quantities, but these will not be reported on a stool test unless they are asked for. It has been reported that as the stool passes through the sigmoid colon, there are chemicals secreted that might decrease the candida numbers as the stool passes through the rectum. The stool stains, of course, have not been quantified, because the illness has not been recognized by the general medical community. In other words, it is a catch-22. In order to prove the illness, some of these things need to be quantified; but since the illness is not believed, any fungal organism seen on a stain is usually considered normal—no matter the quantity of spores present.

Third, since there has been very little scientific information about COS presented to primary-care physicians, relatively few physicians are aware of the information that *is* available that supports the reality of this syndrome. The studies that have been done are not widely published and, in some cases, not believed. Fortunately, as previously stated, there are a number of prominent doctors who recognize and treat this syndrome.

The Evidence

A most impressive trial was conducted by Dr. Carroll Jessop. At the CFS International Conference in 1989, Dr. Jessop reported that of 11,000 patients suffering from chronic fatigue syndrome, 84 percent responded favorably to oral Nizoral and a diet restricting simple sugars and alcohol.[7] An incredible reduction of symptoms was seen in these patients over a 3- to 12-month period. Moreover, in September of 1987, 685 of the 11,000 patients were on disability; but after treatment in April of 1989, only 12 of the 11,000 patients remained on disability. In these patients, chronic candidiasis was suggested by predisposing symptoms: 80 percent of all patients had recurrent antibiotic treatment as a child, adolescent or adult. Sugar-laden diets or alcohol abuse prior to the onset of chronic fatigue syndrome was seen in 95 percent of patients. Other than the obvious fatigue and myalgias, other symptoms such as headaches, irritable bowel syndrome, vaginitis and PMS were very common in these patients. The bottom line is that the symptoms were classic and the results were impressive.

Further support for Dr. Jessop's findings can be obtained through the International Health Foundation in Jackson, Tennessee. Its founder, Dr. William Crook, has written several books including *Tired—So Tired! and the Yeast Connection*. In this book, he cites the following medical studies that document and lend support to COS being a valid syndrome:

1. A 1994 *Journal of Allergy and Clinical Immunology* article published the results of a double-blind placebo-controlled Belgian study revealing that 80 percent of fatigued patients receiving Nizoral improved, whereas 20 percent that received the placebo improved.

2. In 1999, in Virginia, similar improvements were seen in chronic asthma patients with dermatophytosis of the feet (athlete's foot) after treatment with Diflucan. (Note: Many allergists successfully use Diflucan to treat difficult asthma conditions.)

3. Both autism and ADD have responded to antifungal treatment and diet.

4. Endometriosis, interstitial cystitis, psoriasis, bipolar illness, depression and even MS have responded to the same therapy. All this sounds very compelling, and you may ask, "Why are some in the medical community resistant to these findings?" First, most clinicians are not even aware of the information, and if they were privy to such findings, medical curiosity would prompt them at least to try one of the protocols to help their suffering patients. Second, the Dismukes study (outlined below), a single double-blind trial, seemed to dispute the existence of the yeast overgrowth syndrome and its treatment.[8]

The Dismukes Study

As reported in a 1990 *New England Journal of Medicine* article, selected women with typical symptoms of COS were treated with either Nystatin or placebo. The results of the study did not show any significant difference between the control and treated group and, therefore, based upon this one trial, many in the medical establishment dismissed the whole syndrome as unproven. However, many rebuttals to this conclusion were written by physicians who had seen their patients improve dramatically with appropriate treatments.[9]

There are many drugs tested by pharmaceutical companies and/or medical schools that in one double-blind setting have not been shown to be effective statistically. However, follow-up studies using this same medication actually proved the effectiveness of the medication and, thus, reversed the original study findings. Fosamax is one such example. I have seen one early study that failed to show the drug effective in preventing hip fractures. However, virtually every trial since then has proven Fosamax to improve both bone density and prevent hip fractures. Is this a double standard? Don't the candida overgrowth syndrome findings discussed above deserve more attention?

The Dismukes study did not follow the low-sugar Truss protocol. Though Nystatin was used, the diet was not followed. As has been stated, one will not improve over time without an appropriate diet. Dr. W. A. Schrader stated in his response to the negative article in the *NEJM*: "There is practically no hope of successful treatment of this problem without dietary restrictions."[10] Dr. Dennis Remington, in his letter, summarizes it this way: "I would like to recommend that any researcher who evaluates the Truss protocol use the Truss protocol."[11]

CANDIDA AND THE IMMUNOLOGIC RESPONSE

The body's immune response to candida may be the primary reason for the somewhat mysterious symptoms, unless one entertains immune T-cell sensitivity. A candidal allergic mechanism is described elegantly by Dr. R. E. Cater, who attempts to explain that CFS immune dysregulation is very similar to the candidal immune response. The author's explanation of T-cell suppression and reduced production of NK cells and T cells is well documented. It sheds light on the multisystem, nonspecific symptoms observed in COS. The author further elaborates that COS may be a predisposition to CFS, noting that similar immune effects are seen in both patient types:

> Reduced function of cytotoxic T cells and of natural killer cells, as well as interferon reduction, may be important predisposing factors for viral reactivation to take place. By its suppression of T-cell function and consequently of cytotoxic lymphocytic function, NK-cell function and interferon production, chronic Candidiasis of the intestinal mucosa and other mucous membranes may be important predisposing factors, and in some cases, a necessary precursor for the expression of chronic fatigue syndrome.[12]

If this knowledgeable investigator and many others have no problem with the existence of this illness, then physicians should at least consider it in their patients. Why shouldn't they? The treatment is rather benign, but the reward is potentially very beneficial.

MY TREATMENT

If I suspect that someone fits the COS description or if it is obvious by their history that they certainly have the syndrome, I perform an oral swab of their mouth as a screen after a symptom score sheet has been completed. The problem concerning this wet prep of the oral cavity is that it is simply a screen—most people have some yeast at this site as a part of their normal flora. If in doubt, a questionnaire is given.

Once the history, questionnaire and/or the screen are positive, I then give a loading, or challenge, dose of 200 milligrams of Diflucan the first day, followed by 7 to 10 days of 100 milligrams a day on successive days; or I simply give a two- to three-week treatment of either Nizoral or Nystatin.

If the patient improves on the prescribed regimens, then I ask them to return for further instructions in order to follow up on a more comprehensive treatment plan:

1. Acidophilus, Lactinex or a combination probiotic supplement is given.
2. Following the initial 10 days, I prescribe Nystatin tablets three or four times a day for at least four to eight weeks.
3. A diet low in sugar, starches and sometimes mold-containing foods is strongly recommended. Without this diet, the treatment will, in most instances, be worthless.
4. When appropriate, allergy testing and desensitization to TOE (which are considered human yeast) are undertaken.

Discussion

The loading, or challenge, dose of Diflucan kills sufficient yeast to reveal a significant improvement in symptoms in as little as four hours. However, one must be concerned about a Herxheimer's reaction, which may be a result of the immune response to kill off organisms and clear off the end products. This treatment is quite incredible and is similar to relief seen by the use of ibuprofen or Naproxen to treat viral or flu symptoms—the difference being that Diflucan relief lasts days, not hours. This response then is strongly suggestive that a fungal organism is the etiology of the illness.

Consider these points: Over 25 percent of all intestinal bacteria are normal flora; 95 to 99 percent of them are anaerobic and, therefore, are important in digestion and homeostatic functions of the gut. However, these friendly critters also are sensitive to broad-spectrum antibiotics, and large parts of their populations are eliminated as a result. Of course, when this occurs, aggressive growth of organisms such as candida is made possible. In many individuals, the organisms simply regrow their flora and do not succumb to COS. However, it is my experience and the experience of many clinicians that people who are allergy patients are especially at risk. It would make common sense to replenish these cohabitants as one rids the intestines of candida. I do not believe, and neither has it been demonstrable in clinical studies, that intake of probiotics alone is curative. It is necessary that probiotics be combined with antifungals. There are those who believe that it is extremely bad practice not to use probiotics when prescribing broad-spectrum antibiotics such as penicillins, tetracyclines, cephalosporins, quinolone and sulfa medications. As I will discuss later, macrolides are much less likely to induce a candida overgrowth syndrome.

Diflucan, in my opinion, is by far the best drug for this syndrome for the following reasons:

- Diflucan is a most powerful and specific agent designed by Pfizer to eradicate fungal organisms—by far its widest use being that against candida.
- Diflucan is considered the most powerful anticandidal product available.
- Diflucan is almost completely absorbed from the intestines, causing blood levels similar to those of IV injections. This excellent absorption occurs with or without food.
- Diflucan diffuses easily into major bodily fluids including saliva and vaginal secretions and, of course, back into the intestinal tract.

- Diflucan is extremely safe—even in higher doses—but some drug interactions can occur. I would be very careful about interaction with Coumadin, and would be sensitive to the package insert concerning other drug interactions such as certain other antifungals, macrolide antibiotics, statin drugs and the like. Diflucan should not be used during pregnancy.
- Of the thousands of dosages that I have administered to patients, I have seen one, perhaps two, side effects of the medication. A great advantage of Diflucan is that one loading, or challenge, dose can give rapid (within hours) and prolonged (even several days) of relief. Its half-life is approximately 30 hours, but this varies with age groups.

Nystatin is an antifungal medicine that is both fungistatic (stops growth of fungus) and fungicidal (kills fungus)—its action being probably dose-related. It has several great advantages:

- It is not absorbed from the GI tract and, therefore, side effects are rare. Few, if any, systemic reactions have been reported; therefore, it can be used to cleanse the GI tract of candida overgrowth and infections without producing appreciable side effects.
- It can be safely combined with broad-spectrum antibiotics to reduce unwanted yeast multiplication.
- Very little resistance, if any, has occurred with candida.
- It is inexpensive.
- It can be taken over a long period of time to suppress and prevent yeast overgrowth.
- It can be used initially and continually if Diflucan is too expensive and will not be covered by the patient's insurance.

• I strongly recommend it for adults or children who can swallow tablets. This formulation is inexpensive, and it is much easier to take and to put in one's purse or pocket to take later in the day with meals.

A few disadvantages of Nystatin do exist:

• It is not good to take in suspension form since dextrose—a sugar—is one of its inactive ingredients. Since yeast feeds on sugars, it is probably somewhat counterproductive.
• It is not as powerful as Diflucan or other more expensive antifungal agents.
• When given to children, one should use a powder formulation, which may not be easily obtainable from certain pharmacies.

What about the antifungals, Nizoral and Sporanox? Both Nizoral and Sporanox will kill yeast, but their potency and side-effect profile somewhat limit their use, in my opinion. Nizoral specifically has potential side effects beyond 12 to 14 days of use, and I prescribe it only for that length of time. Sporanox may be safer, but it lacks the efficacy of Diflucan and Nizoral for candida specifically. Some physicians who treat COS prefer Nizoral over Diflucan and then will follow the treatment regimen with Nystatin. When used, Nizoral will be ineffective if used with H2 blockers such as Tagamet, Zantac or proton pump inhibitors such as Prilosec and Prevacid. They will prevent the drug from being absorbed and thereby reduce its bioavailability. When Diflucan, for some reason, is not a therapeutic choice, Nizoral and Sporanox are acceptable; but because both drugs have a significant list of potential drug interactions, physicians should be very careful with their use.

Antibiotics

Obviously, the primary initiating risk factor in COS is the use of broad-spectrum antibiotics such as penicillins, tetracyclines, cephalosporins and quinolones. Especially at risk are those patients who are treated for the ulcer-producing organism, *H. pylori*, with multiple antibiotics and powerful acid blockers. Sometimes these antibiotics are called killer-cillins because of their powerful effects. If I use these drugs in what I think is a susceptible patient, I commonly also give a probiotic such as acidophilus, or I suggest the patient eat yogurt or buttermilk.

Preferably, when antibiotics for the respiratory tract are needed, I prefer the macrolide antibiotics, which include erythromycin, Biaxin, Zithromax or Dynabac. These antibiotics primarily eradicate only gram-positive organisms and in large part spare most gram-negative and anaerobic organisms; thus, one doesn't eradicate large populations of friendly bacteria in the gut. For urinary tract infections, I feel that Macrodantin, which concentrates primarily in the urine, is a first-line antibiotic.

CONCLUSION

If gastrointestinal problems aren't resolved with medications,
think yeast.
If chronic fatigue persists and a diagnosis can't be found,
think yeast.
If anxiety, depression or brain fog isn't helped by appropriate treatment,
consider yeast.
If migraine headaches continue in spite of therapy,
think yeast.

If sexual difficulties and recurring vaginitis occur, *think yeast.*

CHAPTER 7

BRAIN FATIGUE

Depression/Anxiety, Bipolar Illness, Sleep Apnea, Chronic Pain, Stress and Addiction

Unless we receive into us that which is above us, we will not be able to cope with that which is around us.

JACK TAYLOR

There is no doubt that the brain plays a central role in the quality of life and how a person feels. The following fatigue-inducing conditions are all caused by a brain chemical dysfunction of some sort:

- Depression/anxiety
- Bipolar illness
- Sleep apnea
- Chronic pain

• Stress
• Addiction

DEPRESSION/ANXIETY

The number one disability worldwide is depression. The number one symptom of depression is fatigue. It is not just a feeling; it is a biochemical process. In some patients, fatigue and body aches may signal depression. In many cases of clinical depression, one can use the measure of fatigue to see how the patient is responding to antidepressants and psychotherapy.

The classic signs, or symptoms, of depression are listed below, using the famous acronym "SADAFACES."

Symptoms of Depression

Sleep—insomnia
Appetite—increases or decreases
Dysthymia (bad mood)
Anhedonia (lack of pleasure)
Fatigue
Agitation
Concentration problems
Esteem—low self- or guilt
Suicidal thoughts

Anxiety, which may be defined as a foreboding uneasiness about the present or future, is also a biochemical process and will eventually produce fatigue. Much of the time, anxiety and depression occur together, but there are about 20 to 25 percent of depressed people who state that they are flat depressed—meaning without energy and without anxiety.

Chemical Imbalance

Without getting overly technical, the three chemicals that are related to depression and anxiety are norepinephrine (NE), serotonin (SE) and dopamine (DA). When there is a decrease in any of these brain chemicals, then depression and anxiety can result. When serotonin is low—causing symptoms (in addition to depression) of insomnia, anxiety and sometimes panic—an SSRI, Effexor or Remeron is very helpful. Effexor especially improves both NE and SE and may be most advantageous. But if a patient has flat depression, then we consider that patient as probably having low norepinephrine and dopamine levels in the brain. In this type of patient, Wellbutrin is the drug of choice in my clinic. Fatigue is a symptom of either type of depression, and when the depression and/or the anxiety is resolved, the fatigue will remit.

The number one symptom of depression is fatigue. It is not just a feeling; it is a biochemical process.

Some neurophysiologists believe that abnormal cortisol—a stress hormone secreted by the adrenal glands that produces a profound effect on the brain—is a culprit in fatigue and depression. There are other researchers who believe that low dopamine and high serotonin in certain areas—especially the basal ganglia—cause fatigue.[1] It is probably a combination of these factors. Drugs are now being developed that may influence the cortisol and brain chemical balance, and at least in early studies, they appear to be very effective.

Other thought-provoking studies on depression suggest that brain chemical imbalance (such as SE, NE or DA) may be the result of, and not the cause of, depression. Steven Stahl, the well-known psychopharmacologist at the University of California in San Diego, has published some very important facts on fatigue and depression. Fatigue is so closely related to depression that the number of days spent in bed is a good indicator of the severity of the depression. Dr. Stahl also points out that in the brain it is low norepinephrine and dopamine rather than serotonin that correlate with fatigue. Therefore, a drug that increases these neurochemicals will cause an energy increase, as is usually the case with Wellbutrin.[2]

Remedies

Natural remedies that are often used in depression include St. John's Wort and SAM-e. Research has not proven their effectiveness, and they do have side effects, so make sure to talk to your physician before taking them. Exercise, however, has been conclusively proven to diminish depression. A study at Duke University found that depressed people who exercised 30 minutes a day, three days a week, improved as rapidly as those taking the antidepressant Zoloft. In addition, they had a lower rate of relapse. One explanation could be that during exercise, the brain releases endorphins, which are neurotransmitters that cause a feeling of well-being.

Remember that depression can be secondary to other illnesses. For example, heart attack or coronary artery bypass patients often have depression due to their disease process, and the same is true for CFS and FMS patients. The bottom line is that if treatment resolves your depression and anxiety, but the fatigue persists, then further investigation is obviously required.

BIPOLAR ILLNESS

People who suffer from bipolar illness, a genetically induced brain disorder (sometimes called manic-depressive disorder), have fatigue as a major symptom. Fatigue during the depressive part of the illness is understandable, but the manic phase also is fatiguing. This euphoric, insomnia-resulting, agitating phase has nervous fatigue as its major symptom in many people. Nervous fatigue is similar to the excititoneurotoxicity found in CFS. Since manics respond very well to sedatives such as Xanax, Klonopin and barbiturates, there is probably NMDA hypervigilance and down-regulation of GABA (see chapter 3). It also is noteworthy that Lithium and other mood stabilizers dramatically help this neuro-toxic type of fatigue. The bipolar patient can have a double wham-my of fatigue, both in his or her depressive and manic phase.

Bipolar illness is, in my estimation, very easy to treat if the patient will simply take his or her medicine. The medicine usual-ly consists of a mood stabilizer and an antidepressant. The anti-depressant of choice in bipolar illness is Wellbutrin. When I diag-nose a new case of bipolar illness, I usually start the patient on the mood stabilizer first and add Wellbutrin later. Some patients, however, may already be on antidepressants, since even the best psychiatrist can be fooled by the subtle symptoms of the different types of bipolar disease. It is very important to note that when the bipolar patient is in neither a depressive nor manic phase, even psychological testing will not clearly diagnose the condition. The clinician must simply always have this disorder in mind when interviewing patients who have not responded to the typical ther-apies for anxiety and depression.

SLEEP APNEA

A very common cause of fatigue that is poorly recognized by many health-care professionals, but one that can be treated eas-ily most of the time, is sleep apnea. Although sleep apnea is not caused by neural factors, it does have a profound effect on the function of the brain. The fact that deep sleep is important in optimal brain function and energy metabolism can be illustrat-ed by this abnormality. Virtually every patient with significant sleep apnea will have fatigue, but the hallmark of this illness is hypersomnia, or daytime drowsiness. A good night's sleep doesn't resolve the patient's feeling of sleepiness. If sleep apnea sufferers sit still for just a short time, they doze off. This happens because their snoring the previous night prevented them from entering into the deeper stages of sleep, which are necessary for healthful rest. Much of the time, there is an obstruction in the airways that causes apnea (lack of breathing) for a few seconds, thus interrupting the sleep cycle. Some patients will even stop breathing for a few seconds—as many as 60 times in a 90-minute period. Research has shown that obesity plays a role in sleep apnea as well. Many patients find that after losing weight, their snoring diminishes significantly.

In a single night, an individual generally needs five cycles of stages I-V (light to deep) sleep, followed by a REM phase. When snoring and apnea interrupt these cycles, a form of sleeping insomnia occurs. Many people are not even aware that they snore or that they stop breathing, but when they awaken, they generally do not feel rested.

Treatment

Sleep apnea usually can be resolved by a sleep specialist—usually an ear, nose and throat doctor. A lab sleep study is recommended, during which the patient's brain, breathing and heart activity are monitored. Then a definitive diagnosis can be made. A machine called a C-PAP then may be fitted to the patient, and the syndrome will likely be completely resolved. It is amazing how much better the patient will feel after using this device on a nightly basis. At first it may be annoying, but most people can accommodate it.

Case Report

A local businessman complaining of periodic anxiety, weight gain and headaches had been to my office for a number of years.

However, the patient, on one particular visit, was asked if he snored. The answer was yes. I sent him for an evaluation and, indeed, he had sleep apnea and was treated with the C-PAP machine. The improvement in his quality of life was absolutely amazing. He stated that he could concentrate and think better, and the fatigue (which had not been recognized as fatigue due to the other symptoms) had been resolved. His weight decreased and his cholesterol went down, and the use of benzodiazepines was discontinued. I had a very happy patient.

CHRONIC PAIN

Another neurally induced cause of fatigue is chronic pain. Most of the time, the chronic pain is associated with a direct injury to a set of nerves such as that in lumbar or cervical spine injuries. However, sometimes there has been no injury, and the patient has what is called spinal stenosis. This is a narrowing in the spinal canal that compresses the nerves in the cord, thus producing pain. In some people, the compression in the lumbar area (lower back) causes pain upon walking or standing; but while at rest, sitting or lying down, they have no pain.

Pain also can be caused by postherpes neuralgia, which occurs after shingles. This can be resolved through an allergy procedure called histamine neutralization or by medications such as Neurontin, Depakote and Tegretol. Other neurally induced causes of pain include tic douloureux, or facial nerve pain, and pain syndromes due to diabetic neuropathy. Chronic pain syndromes such as arthritis, tendonitis, bursitis and soft-tissue crush injuries can all be sources of fatigue.

Causes

The exact reason for fatigue in chronic pain is not clear. Some believe it is simply due to the interruption of sleep due to pain.

Others believe that it is the lack of homeostasis that ultimately affects cell energy output. Still other clinicians think that the depression that often accompanies chronic pain is the primary mechanism that causes fatigue. Whatever the cause, tiredness is usually seen in chronic pain patients and is probably a combination of all of the above.

Treatment

As previously stated, if neuropathic pain is present, a combination of either Effexor or Wellbutrin, Elavil in low doses at night and sometimes antiseizure drugs such as Neurontin, Depakote or Tegretol are very helpful. Of course, the treatment of insomnia is primary; and if Elavil is not effective, then a GABA agonist such as Ambien, Zanaflex or Klonopin is my choice. Narcotics should be the last resort in cases of severe, unrelenting pain.

As in other fatigue syndromes, exercise, physical therapy and/or massage therapy are helpful. Exercise decreases immune pain mediators, promotes helpful sleep and decreases insulin resistance, which lowers the proinflammatory immune factor TNF-alpha. Therefore, minimal to moderate exercise is extremely useful.

STRESS

Pavlov was the first to describe the role of stress in health and disease. In a fascinating paper in the *New England Journal of Medicine* several years ago, the authors identified several risk factors in the development of viral syndromes such as colds. The major factors were lack of sleep, lack of exercise, poor eating habits, alcohol and stress. The conclusion drawn by the authors was that stress was the most important risk factor of all. In fact, when the individual was under stress, the other factors listed above were more likely to occur.

Notably, stress induces mental fatigue called burnout. Over a period of time, the response to stress is detrimental to the immune system, which contributes to fatigue. In the Old Testament, Solomon gives this salient and truthful observation:

A calm and undisturbed mind and heart are the life and health of the body, but envy, jealousy, and wrath are like rottenness of the bones (Prov. 14:30, *AMP*).

The cells that make up our immune system are basically manufactured in the bone marrow as well as the lymph nodes. In order to keep our bones and our immune system healthy, we must learn how to deal with the stresses that we all face in life.

Spiritual maturity, which comes from trusting in God, praying and developing close relationships with other Christians, also provides a necessary source of strength for withstanding the negative impacts of stress.

Prevention

Prevention of excess stress is, of course, the best antidote. Adequate rest, exercise and healthy eating patterns help us cope with everyday stresses. Spiritual maturity, which comes from trusting in God, praying and developing close relationships with other Christians, also provides a necessary source of strength for withstanding the negative impacts of stress. People who work at resolving conflicts and forgiving others seem to have an easier time letting go of the events and emotions that generate stress in most individuals. The driving forces of self-induced stress—workaholism, compulsive tendencies, perfectionism, guilt and the need for control—are often born from past rejections, resulting in anger. Negative emotions such as anger and fear create a physical response that causes distress to the body and mind.

Case Report

I have attended several mission trips to Brazil where we saw literally thousands of people come to Christ, tens of thousands of people helped through medical and dental services and people miraculously healed by the power of God. During an altar call one night at a fairly large church in Governador Valadares, a middle-aged woman came to the front, crying and weeping. She was completely worn out. People who were observing her and listening to her story might have thought she was overwhelmed by physical, emotional or diseased-induced stress. But that was not the case. She was a woman who felt like it was her job to control everyone's lives and fix everybody's problems. She was failing miserably, and nights of insomnia and days of anxiety had eventually induced depression and burnout. After prayer, the strong suggestion was made that she simply let go and let God handle all of these problems. She only needed to pray for people. Martha, the wife of the minister who led these large teams down to Brazil, commented to me that she was once a person such as this. She had always tried to be a savior for everyone, but she had to release herself into God's care and trust Him to take care of her problems as well as everyone else's problems. Martha then was set free from her problem.

ADDICTION

Addiction: When a person doesn't have something or do something, he or she feels bad; but when the person does have this something or does it, he or she doesn't feel good. In other words, the person has poor quality of life with or without the substance or activity. Addictions can be broken down into two types: (1) substance addictions, and (2) process addictions.

Substance Addictions

The substance addictions are obvious. They include things like alcohol, morphine, cocaine, nicotine, caffeine and food. Yes, I said food. In many cases, the cause of obesity is compulsive eating—the person eats even when not hungry. Compulsive eaters may be bulimic or anorexic, but more commonly they simply love food. According to *Love Hunger: Recover from Food Addiction*, a book written by Frank Minirth, M.D., these people are simply feeding the emptiness and the worthlessness they feel within.[3] This is probably true of all addictions.

Addiction: When a person doesn't have something or do something, he or she feels bad; but when the person does have this something or does it, he or she doesn't feel good.

Process Addictions

In process addictions, there is no chemical involved but instead an activity. These activities may include pornography, gambling or excessive shopping and spending. Although there is no chemical intake, the same neural changes that occur in substance addictions also are present in those that have process addictions. Researchers and clinicians that treat addictions know that low dopamine in the brain is associated with addictive tendencies. Addicted individuals are not driven by common sense or normal cognitive choices. They usually are driven by the pleasure center in the brain. One might say that if you have low dopamine in your brain, your brain is in jail. Not only is there a sadistic driving force that causes an uncomfortable, compulsive feeling in these people, but they also experience varying amounts of fatigue and depression. As addiction continues over time, there is progressive loss of dopamine neurons in the brain, as well as other brain chemicals such as endorphins, enkephalins and serotonin.

Heroin Versus Fast Food

During a small round-table meeting, Dr. Howard Metzmin, an addictionologist in New Orleans, Louisiana, stated that one of the most powerful mood-altering drugs in Western society is fast food. There is no difference in the PET brain scans of an obese person and a heroin addict. In other words, the same deadly loss of dopamine occurs in both. I commented at the meeting that the insulin resistance that causes craving of junk foods filled with sugar, starch and fat probably is chemically directly related to a lack of dopamine in the brain. Dr. Metzmin agreed and stated that the number one treatment for compulsive eating, as well as many other addictions in our society, is the dopamine-enhancing medication Wellbutrin (bupropion). As dopamine concentrations are raised in the brain, the feelings of addiction are decreased. Of course, all of these people would benefit from spiritual and psychological counseling to help overcome addiction problems, because the answer is not found in only a pill. Wellbutrin is an adjunct to spiritual and emotional healing.

I also emphasize to compulsive eaters who are fatigued that they may be suffering from yeast overgrowth, because yeast will induce a craving for sugar and simple starches. Therefore, a trial of the antifungal Diflucan also may be in order. I have actually had patients return to my office and say that the desire for sugar stopped after they took Diflucan and probiotics (see chapter 6).

Case Report

A person can overcome addictions only if he or she really wants to. A young woman with fatigue and obesity once came to my office. There was no special history of illness, no family history of major disease, and no medications were being taken that could explain her feelings of weakness and shakiness. Somewhat puzzled, I asked her if she ingested an abundance of starchy or sugary foods. To my amazement, she said that she ate a sack of flour almost every afternoon after work. This compulsive, addictive habit was the source of her poor quality of life. I suggested to her that she must discontinue this behavior. The patient never returned to the clinic. If she returned to my clinic today, I would start her on Wellbutrin and Avandia, and I would search for a possible yeast overgrowth in her intestines. People like this *can* be helped.

Conclusion

Brain fatigue is common in our society and manifests itself in the various ways listed above, as well as many more. We live in a stressful world that takes its toll on our minds and bodies. As long as we are alive on Earth, we won't get rid of all the physical and emotional stresses that contribute to brain fatigue. But what we do have is God's powerful presence and the wise counsel of His Word to guide us through our lives. God's Word will help keep our minds and bodies healthy.

You will keep in perfect peace him whose mind is steadfast,
because he trusts in you.

ISAIAH 26:3

Thou wilt keep him in perfect peace, whose mind is stayed on thee:
because he trusteth in thee. Trust ye in the LORD for ever:
for in the LORD JEHOVAH is everlasting strength.

ISAIAH 26:3-4, KJV

CHAPTER 8

IMMUNE FATIGUE

Allergies, Environmental Toxins and Chemical Sensitivities, Pernicious Anemia, Infections, and Polymyalgia Rheumatica of the Elderly

The two basic processes of the immune system are that of protection and repair. God put an incredible memory inside the protective part of the immune system, whereby it can detect and kill approximately 200,000 invaders. A main function of the immune system's job is to distinguish self from nonself. That which is nonself is destroyed; that which is self is protected. This is the protective part of our immunity. The repair system, though complicated, is straightforward; and it basically helps put back together cells that are destroyed through injury or illness.

When an invader (anything that can harm the body) comes into contact with the body, the immune system detects it and describes and imprints upon itself the nature of the enemy. That message is sent back to cells called lymphocytes, and they begin to manufacture antibodies. These antibodies are stored and then released to search and destroy when confronted again by that same invader. The human immune response also consists of cells that simply engulf and destroy these invaders.

God put an incredible memory inside the protective part of the immune system, whereby it can detect and kill approximately 200,000 invaders.

This complicated system is monitored by chemical messengers called cytokines. They carry very powerful messages from the brain to the immune system. When they are functioning in a normal way, they are extremely effective in the overall protective system. But when they overreact, the attack on the enemy (toxins) results in destruction of the host (healthy tissue). This incredible protective system includes five classes of immunoglobulins—IgG, IgM, IgA, IgE and IgD. These antibodies are essential to immune health. The IgG antibodies are part of our long-term immune memory. The IgM antibodies are part of the quick-response system. The IgA antibodies protect the respiratory and GI tracts. The IgE antibodies are associated with allergies. The function of IgD antibodies is unknown. Common fatiguing illnesses that cause, or are caused by, immune system dysfunction include:

- Allergies
- Environmental toxins and chemical sensitivities
- Pernicious anemia
- Infections
- Polymyalgia rheumatica of the elderly

ALLERGIES

Allergies are the result of an overreaction of the immune system to biological antigens that are generally benign. For example, ragweed, tree pollen and grass pollen are not injurious to the body; but some individuals' immune systems think they are. In the process, certain chemical mediators such as histamine are released and cause airway congestion, itching and swelling. The immune system's attack on these harmless invaders can adversely affect virtually every system of the body. Allergic diseases include asthma, rhinitis, urticaria, atopic dermatitis and food allergies, to name just a few.

Some common allergens include:

- Chemicals
- Tree pollen
- Mold
- Weeds
- Grass
- Animal hair

The extent of your symptoms is related to the amount of allergen to which the tissue is exposed. This is the concept of allergic load. The greater the amount of exposure to these benign biologic invaders, the more likely one is to experience the symptoms listed below:

- Asthma
- Sneezing
- Conjunctivitis (itchy, red eyes)
- Intestinal problems
- Itching
- Rash

· Nasal congestion

· Fatigue

Fatigue is one of the major symptoms that results from allergic load. The mechanism whereby fatigue is caused by exposure to allergens has at least three explanations:

1. An overactive immune system requires constant vigilance for which extra energy is continually required. The load on the mitochondria in the cells might be viewed as an automobile continually traveling 100 miles an hour without any stops. This necessitates more calories, minerals, vitamins and nutrients to fuel the cells' activities.

2. Because of this hypervigilance of the immune system, proinflammatory cytokines are released throughout the body, inducing aching and fatigue themselves, much like when one has influenza. Fortunately, this release is not as exaggerated as with a viral infection, and the fatigue is not nearly as severe. Remember that it is not the invader that causes the aching and fatigue directly, but it is the body's immune response that causes these symptoms.

3. Research has indicated that there are some differences between the brain of an allergic patient and the brain of a nonallergic patient. During an allergy attack, the central nervous system is usually involved and some brain mechanisms are compromised, producing what one may call neural fatigue. Insomnia can be one result of this process, since postnasal drip, cough, congestion and fever can inhibit sleep.

There is no doubt that one's quality of life is affected with prolonged allergic response. The following questionnaire will help you and your doctor determine the extent to which your allergies are a problem:

Quality-of-Life Questionnaire

Name _____

Date _____

For each item listed, indicate how much trouble your allergy symptoms have caused you in the last week. Please use the following scale:

0 = Not troubled
1 = Hardly troubled at all
2 = Somewhat troubled
3 = Moderately troubled
4 = Quite troubled
5 = Very troubled
6 = Extremely troubled

Sleep Problems:
1. Difficulty falling asleep   0   1   2   3   4   5   6
2. Waking up during the night   0   1   2   3   4   5   6
3. Not having a good night's sleep   0   1   2   3   4   5   6

General Symptoms:
1. Fatigue   0   1   2   3   4   5   6
2. Thirst   0   1   2   3   4   5   6
3. Reduced productivity 0   1   2   3   4   5   6
4. Tiredness   0   1   2   3   4   5   6
5. Poor concentration   0   1   2   3   4   5   6

Continued on next page

Continued from previous page

6. Headache	0	1	2	3	4	5	6
7. Feeling worn out	0	1	2	3	4	5	6

Practical Problems:

1. Having to carry tissues or a handkerchief	0	1	2	3	4	5	6
2. Having to rub your nose/eyes	0	1	2	3	4	5	6
3. Having to blow your nose often	0	1	2	3	4	5	6

Nasal Symptoms:

1. Stuffed/blocked nose	0	1	2	3	4	5	6
2. Runny nose	0	1	2	3	4	5	6
3. Sneezing	0	1	2	3	4	5	6
4. Postnasal drip	0	1	2	3	4	5	6

Eye Symptoms:

1. Itchy eyes	0	1	2	3	4	5	6
2. Watery eyes	0	1	2	3	4	5	6
3. Sore eyes	0	1	2	3	4	5	6

Activity Limitation:

Identify three activities limited by symptoms in the past week.

Activity 1	0	1	2	3	4	5	6

Specify activity _____

Activity 2	0	1	2	3	4	5	6

Specify activity _____

Continued from previous page

Activity 3   0 1 2 3 4 5 6
Specify activity_____

Emotional Symptoms:
How often during the last week have you been troubled by these emotions as a result of your allergy symptoms?

1. Frustration	0 1 2 3 4 5 6
2. Impatience or restlessness	0 1 2 3 4 5 6
3. Irritability	0 1 2 3 4 5 6
4. Embarrassment	0 1 2 3 4 5 6

All in all, allergy patients suffer with more than just runny noses. Numerous studies have shown that children who suffer from allergies have decreased test scores and do worse in school than nonallergic children. Adult allergy patients usually have lower productivity in the workplace.

Case Report

A 43-year-old physician complaining of a 30-year history of postnasal drip, nasal congestion, frequent sinus infections and fatigue came to my office. When talking to patients and speaking to various groups, he noted that he continually had to clear his throat due to the increased amount of postnasal drip. He had been on periodic antibiotics and had tried virtually every available treatment for allergies. I started him on allergy shots after appropriate testing and within several months he began experiencing welcome relief from his nasal and sinus symptoms as well as from the years of silent fatigue. He continued on immunotherapy for approximately five years and has continued to be in remission from these symptoms. At age 54, he states that he feels better overall than he did 30 years ago.

Treatment

Avoidance of allergens should be the first approach to treatment of allergies. Allergic symptoms also can be treated with medications. Antihistamines such as Allegra (choice antihistamine of the *Medical Letter*[1]), Zyrtec (which helps the late phase response as described earlier) and Clarinex (which has been shown in research to inhibit cytokine production) can be very helpful in alleviating fatigue. The addition of decongestants such as Sudafed, Pan Mist and the like may be helpful also. Nasal steroids are effective for congestion, but they are not particularly helpful in fatigue. NSAIDS such as Advil and Naprosyn can help calm down the inflammatory response and can be helpful in relieving the tiredness.

The history of medicine has documented the association between air and water pollution and an increase in allergies and chemical sensitivity.

The most impressive medications for fatigue are cortisone-type drugs. However, one should not use these medicines for more than a few days, due to adverse side effects. These drugs are more suited for other conditions for a longer period of time. Their use for allergies is only acceptable for the short-term.

Immunotherapy is the administration of allergy shots, which are given to certain individuals who cannot avoid the allergens they are sensitive to and do not respond well to the other allergy medications listed. Immunotherapy is the most consistent and effective way to treat allergic fatigue. The combination of immunotherapy and other medications, in my experience, has been very effective in treating CFS. FMS has not responded as well, so I usually do not recommend immunotherapy unless the patient has allergies that do not respond to other measures.

ENVIRONMENTAL TOXINS AND CHEMICAL SENSITIVITIES

Environmental toxins and chemicals have been blamed for a number of illnesses that afflict mankind. Connective-tissue diseases, lung disease, various skin diseases and even cancer are some of the sicknesses that are related to environmental exposure and toxicity. Of course, people who are allergy sufferers are usually hypersensitive to toxins and chemicals in the environment. Some patients in particular cannot deal with chemicals and toxins and succumb to a chronic fatigue-type illness, while others may be exposed to the same chemicals and not succumb to obvious disease. There is a clear genetic predisposition to the sensitivities mentioned.

Exposure to Toxins

The Industrial Revolution produced many incredible inventions, but with it came an increase in inhalant allergies. In Japan, for example, few were allergic to mountain cedar pollen until the rapid growth of factories and the careless disposal of chemical waste. The history of medicine has documented the association between air and water pollution and an increase in allergies and chemical sensitivity.

Chemical solvents, formaldehydes and oil-based paints are a few examples of indoor pollutants that have adversely affected many patients. Other sources of exposure to toxic substances are found in homes, automobiles, clothes, food, water, volatile solvents, pesticides, herbicides, PCBs and metals. Most exposure comes through inhalation of vapors and dust, ingestion of chemicals in food and water, and skin contact with clothing and dyes.

Well-known examples of chemical exposure and its detrimental effects on human health are that of Agent Orange exposure in the Vietnam War and that of chemical exposure that occurred in the Iraqi campaign of 1991 (Gulf War Syndrome). The detrimental effects were specific to certain groups of men and women who apparently were genetically susceptible. The degree of illness is generally dependent upon the concentration of the poison with which a person has contact. However, some genetically sensitive individuals are severely effected by even low levels of exposure.

Toxic Effects

Environmental toxins and chemicals primarily effect two areas in the human body: the immune system and the nervous system, respectively called immunotoxicity and neurotoxicity. When toxic chemicals interact with the immune system, there are three possible undesirable effects:

1. There is an immediate or delayed hypersensitive reaction.
2. There may be immune suppression.
3. There may be immune activation.

When the immune system is adversely effected—no matter the mechanism of action—disease and certainly fatigue will result.

The second major system that is effected is the nervous system. The following neurotoxic effects are listed in the diagnosis code book in medical offices:

- Personality changes, including irritability and social withdrawal
- Mental changes, which include problems with recent memory, concentration and mental slowness
- Sleep disturbances

- Chronic fatigue
- Headaches
- Sexual dysfunction
- Numbness in hands and/or feet
- Recognition that there has been a loss of mental function

Most clinicians believe that it requires a relatively high concentration of toxins to produce changes in the central nervous system. However, ongoing exposure to low levels of chemicals, which may go unnoticed over time, can cause neurotoxicity. Some individuals may simply detox these chemicals in their bodies, and sickness does not result. However, because of genetic predisposition, some people may subtly develop various illnesses due to low-level exposure. The genetic variation between individuals results in different degrees of biologic, metabolic and detoxification responses to the same medication or environmental pollutant. In other words, some people can metabolize certain chemicals and others cannot. These patients have multiple chemical sensitivity (MCS), implying that they are at risk with exposure to low levels of toxicity.

In the medical community, there has been skepticism of multiple chemical sensitivity and its effect on the body, in particular on the brain. SPECT scans, which are special metabolic scans of the brain, have shown evidence of neurotoxicity in 90 percent of MCS patients. These abnormalities are compatible with the cognitive symptoms that are frequently reported by patients.[2]

The same journal reported that SPECT scans were performed before and after blinded exposure to very low concentrations of relevant chemicals. This study showed a high degree of neurotoxicity in MCS patients, and it was not characteristic of SPECT features of psychiatric illness. In other words, these patients were thought to have psychiatric disease, but the SPECT scans proved otherwise.

The symptoms that MCS patients report in addition to allergic symptoms are those that parallel CFS symptoms, which obviously include fatigue. I believe that the basic reason why people succumb to fatigue in chemically induced syndromes is the effect on mitochondria, which are the energy-producing factories of our cells.

Treatment

Fortunately, God, the creator, placed within us incredible enzyme systems to rid the body of poisons. When these systems are overwhelmed, however, sickness, fatigue and even death can result. The diagnosis of chemical sensitivities is not difficult, but it should be done by a competent environmental medicine doctor or an industrial toxicologist. Indeed, the average primary-care physician is not well trained in the area of chemical toxicology, and therefore this important cause of fatigue may be overlooked. An MCS diagnosis can be made using a 24-hour urine test, hair analysis, special immunochemical tests, and skin, or provocation, tests. Provocation tests with DMSO or DMBA are superior. If you have fatigue and allergies, and you tend to be sensitive to certain smokes, vapors and chemicals, and a clear diagnosis has not been made, consider multiple chemical sensitivities.

The treatment for MCS includes ingesting vitamins and minerals, especially zinc and magnesium, which are key cofactors in inducing enzyme systems to rid the body of toxins. Another method of detoxing the body is by frequenting a sauna. The sweating that results is a way of excreting chemicals from the body. Chelation therapy also is a very important way to rid the body of metal toxicities such as mercury and lead. Chelation consists of delivering certain medicinals that latch onto the toxic chemicals and then are naturally excreted from the body. High doses of vitamin C can be helpful because that vitamin is a natural chelator. In specific patients, the use of antidepressants such as Effexor, Wellbutrin and Elavil also can be beneficial, as they improve brain function.

Mold Toxins

When water damage occurs in a dwelling, certain toxic molds can begin growing. The same can occur in basements where water and moisture collect. Molds thrive in moist environments. Not only can they be allergenic to individuals, but also they can liberate other toxins, which can induce significant illness and fatigue. The reason molds release toxins is that there is a competition for the microenvironment with other molds and bacteria. In releasing toxins, they kill the other inhabitants of this environment so that they can thrive.

Some individuals are unfortunately poisoned by these toxic molds, and their symptoms are typically that of fatigue, brain fog, listlessness, irritable bowel syndrome and cognitive dysfunction. These are virtually the same symptoms as chronic fatigue syndrome. Since the toxic effects of molds can mimic other diseases, it is important to keep this in mind as a possibility when treatments for other illnesses are not effective.

The only reliable treatment for mold-induced illness is to remove and destroy the mold from the building, which sometimes means removing part of the dwelling. Some molds of the genus *Stachybotrys* are so dangerous and life-threatening that when discovered, the house and everything inside must be burned. This mold cannot be eradicated by normal fungicidal methods, so fire is the only recourse.

Case Report 1. A 42-year-old pastor's wife with a history of worsening inhalant allergies as well as hoarseness, coldness, fatigue and alopecia came to my office. She had been diagnosed with hypothyroidism. She had been experiencing increasing sinus symptoms—especially after moving into a new parsonage—

and had developed fibromyalgia with classic trigger points on her physical exam. She was given appropriate allergy medicine as well as antibiotics for her sinusitis. However, she returned complaining of further sinus symptoms. A nasal swab revealed numerous yeast organisms. She was treated with Diflucan and improved somewhat. She also started on an allergy regimen. Her fatigue and quality of life again worsened until she and her husband discovered mold-type organisms growing in an area of the parsonage that had had water damage. Health officials confirmed the presence of toxin-producing mold and an effort was made to eradicate the mold. However, the patient's symptoms did not improve until they moved to another town. The patient endured two sinus surgeries, allergy shots, frequent antibiotics for sinus infections, fungal sinusitis and sarcoidosis—all as a result of an apparent toxic mold. As far as I know, she is now recovering and doing very well.

Case Report 2. A teenage girl was presented at one of our American Academy of Environmental Medicine meetings. She was experiencing fatigue, headaches, dizziness, other neurological symptoms and weakness to the point that she was brought into the meeting in a wheelchair. At the time, she was seeing a psychiatrist for anxiety and depression. This young lady had been very healthy prior to her illness, which had been ongoing for approximately three months. Numerous medical visits, consultations, MRIs, X rays and laboratory tests failed to determine a diagnosis. Chemicals, environmental toxins, chronic fatigue syndrome, fibromyalgia and other possible causes of her illness were discussed at the meeting. However, there was one clear-cut historical fact: Water damage had occurred to her house a few months prior to her illness. The medical audience offered several suggestions, one of which was that the family investigate possible toxic mold. The family greatly appreciated our input and decided to take steps to rule out toxic mold.

The meeting's moderator, Dr. Lieberman, sent all the participants a follow-up letter several months later. Mold had been found in the home, and the mold was found to be more toxic than originally expected: it necessitated extensive home reconstruction and replacement of the walls, bricks on the rear of the house, carpeting, ceiling and furniture. During this reconstruction, the patient had moved out of the house and made an incredible improvement in her health. She was able to start walking with crutches and renewed her interest in some old activities. She finished the school year with a 4.0 GPA, and her health continued to improve. Her mother, in the follow-up letter, thanked the doctors for their input and for the many people who were praying for her daughter.

This is a powerful reminder to all physicians and health-care providers that illnesses that appear to be other diseases may actually have an environmental cause. If the patient is not responding to therapy that should improve their health, then other diagnoses must be sought.

The following lists the treatment for mold toxicity:

1. Remove the mold or move the person out of the dwelling.
2. Treat with immunotherapy.
3. Treat with appropriate antihistamines and decongestants.
4. If all of the above fail, order a FACT test. If the results are positive, order cholestyramine, Welchol plus Actos or Avandia.

PERNICIOUS ANEMIA

An insidious and frequently overlooked cause of fatigue in middle-aged and older adults is pernicious anemia. A more accurate name for this illness would be low B12 syndrome. The typical symptoms include:

- Fatigue
- Decreased mental concentration with eventual dementia
- Paresthesia (numbness)
- Anemia with larger than normal red blood cells
- Inflammation of the tongue and mouth

Pernicious anemia is generally considered hereditary and is an autoimmune disorder in which certain cells in the stomach that secrete intrinsic factor are destroyed. Intrinsic factor, when released, attaches to ingested vitamin B12 and permits it to be absorbed later in the small intestines. When intrinsic factor is not present, 99 percent of ingested B12 is not absorbed.

Since the body stores B12, it takes a while for the B12 to be depleted. This is God's way of protection when one doesn't eat the necessary B12 foods. B12 is vital for brain, red blood cell, immune and energy mechanisms. Vitamin B12 is present in all foods of animal origin, so a strict vegetarian who avoids all dairy products as well as meat and fish is susceptible to B12 deficiency, although the individual may still have intrinsic factor in his or her stomach. Certain surgeries of the abdomen and stomach also can inhibit B12 absorption and cause a limitation of intrinsic factor secretion. Occasionally, tapeworms, pancreatic insufficiency and severe Crohn's disease can retard B12 absorption.

The normal level of B12 is greater than 212 in blood tests, but I become suspicious when levels lower than 300 are found in those individuals with classic symptoms. If this occurs, I repeat the B12 blood test in one to three months and order a methylmalonic acid test, which is now available from most major laboratories.

When pernicious anemia is diagnosed, a regimen of B12 shots is ordered with loading concentrations early, and eventually 1,000 to 2,000 micrograms are given once a month for maintenance. (I am currently administering oral B12 at 1,000 micrograms per day instead of shots if the patient so desires.)

Case History

A 58-year-old man came to my clinic after hearing that I treated patients with fatigue. Previous physician visits were unfruitful and the patient was beginning to experience some concentration problems, numbness in extremities and some soreness in his mouth. The patient's history revealed a stomach operation many years previously for ulcers, and he had a dumping syndrome requiring him to eat small meals. His fatigue was slow in onset and progressive. A physical exam revealed a mild decrease in sensation in his feet, with no other abnormalities noted. Anemia was not seen in the laboratory test, but atypical large red blood cells were noted. In addition, an abnormal B12 level was found. The patient was started on appropriate B12 shots and totally recovered in a three-month period.

INFECTIONS

All infections can cause fatigue; however, there are several that are sometimes overlooked when searching for a diagnosis in fatigue patients.

Nostril Bacteria Breeding

It is known among infectious-disease experts and other physicians who are interested in occult and chronic infections that people can harbor certain harmful bacteria in their noses. These bacteria—especially the ones that are resistant to particular antibiotics—can cause chronic fatigue. If I suspect nostril bacteria, I will culture the patient's nares. If the culture returns showing a heavy growth of normal upper respiratory flora, this is negative. But if they have one specific bacteria such as staph, strep or even gram-negative bacteria, this must be treated. Depending on the type of bacteria, I use Bactroban applications into the nose three times a day plus other antibiotics if necessary. This is such a simple pro-.cedure, yet it has a profound effect on a patient's well-being—so much so that it should be done on any patient who does not respond to normal therapy.

Occult Infections of the Colon

The colon is known to harbor—as its normal flora—parasites, bacteria and fungi. However, when these bacteria overgrow in certain people, fatigue and other disorders can cause distress. Some organisms may be present because of antibiotic usage, but others are there due to naturally occurring diarrheal diseases such as salmonella, shigella and so on.

Case History. A young woman called me in desperation because she had been fatigued for many months. She had loose stools, gas and occasional blood in her stool. At times she had brain fog and insomnia. Her family believed she was psychosomatic. Two other physicians had diagnosed her with irritable bowel syndrome. After a conversation on the phone, during which I found out she had been on antibiotics, I diagnosed pseudomembranous enterocolitis. I began her on 250 milligrams of Flagyl three times a day for 10 days, as well as cholestyramine. Within two days, she had greatly improved. Later we found that her lab tests were indeed positive for this organism.

This particular bacteria releases toxins into the system that can cause significant difficulties and is usually more acute than in this patient's case. When a person has had diarrhea over several days, I almost always ask them if they have had a previous dose of antibiotics. If they have, I order appropriate fecal tests and treat according to the findings. If the patient has a past history of salmonella or shigella, and he or she continues to have loose stools or diarrhea plus fatigue, the physician must consider a symbiotic relationship between those particular bacteria and the body. In some cases, the body quells the acute phase overgrowth but allows the bacteria to continue to grow. This may be, in part, an immune problem. Other colon infections are parasitic in nature. Hidden parasites may be involved in the development of glomerular nephritis, arthropathies and arthritis.

I believe that routine stool analysis done in hospitals does not pick up these occult infections. That is why I generally send a complete stool analysis off to a national lab like Smokey Mountain Labs or Doctors Data. Though expensive, this is an important test to include when one cannot ascertain the cause of fatigue. The infection should be treated according to the results of the culture performed by one of the excellent labs above. In many cases, I immediately start treatment with Flagyl, based on my own empirical knowledge; but to get a definitive diagnosis and treatment plan, the stool cultures mentioned are extremely valuable.

Chronic Sinusitis

When an area of the body, such as the sinuses, is not draining well, it can become like a swamp and become infected. Such is the case in chronic sinusitis. The chief symptoms of sinusitis are chronic postnasal drip, nasal congestion, headaches and fatigue. It is interesting to note that the fluid and debris in the maxillary sinuses have to flow upward in order to drain. Because the sinuses drain easily in a supine position, causing a postnasal drip, some people experience a nighttime cough when in bed. This can be a symptom of allergies as well as sinusitis. Over-the-counter antihistamines taken one hour before bedtime can help alleviate this problem.

Ear, nose and throat doctors are experts at diagnosing sinusitis, because they are trained to read sinus X rays. X rays usually will show any sinus congestion or inflammation. If a patient has severe symptoms and the X ray is not definitive, a CT scan of the sinuses should be ordered. Treatment of sinusitis includes antibiotic therapy for approximately three weeks, supplemented with yogurt or acidophilus to prevent intestinal problems. Decongestants along with guaifenesin will help to drain the sinuses while they are healing. A cortisone dosepack allows the antibiotics to work and decrease inflammation. Cortisone nasal sprays are equally important in the process.

Generally, people with chronic sinusitis also have allergies and/or nasal deviation and polyps. These conditions should be addressed so that they will not recur and compound the infection problem.

Mononucleosis

The Epstein-Barr virus is clearly the cause of mononucleosis, or mono. At one time, it was thought to be the cause of chronic fatigue syndrome. Most of the time, the symptoms are classic and include sore throat, enlarged lymph nodes and acute malaise. They are similar to the symptoms of other infectious illnesses but tend to persist longer. However, there are some patients who will not exhibit the classic symptoms of sore throat and/or enlarged lymph nodes of the neck; instead, they will only succumb to the weakness and fatigue. The infection usually lasts from two to four weeks, but it is more prolonged in older patients. It is normal for patients to feel tired for months after the illness.

Diagnosis is made by a blood test to determine an excess of antibodies to the Epstein-Barr virus and an elevated white blood cell (lymphocyte) count. If the IgM part of the viral titer is positive, then mononucleosis can be diagnosed. However, the IgG antibodies mean absolutely nothing for acute mononucleosis. The IgG positive titers primarily mean that the immune system has seen the virus and conquered it earlier in life—one has actually had mononucleosis and the body has dealt with it. I test some patients with a mono spot lab test, which can be easily done in the office, but it must be remembered that the mono spot may not become positive until after the first week of the illness.

Since there is no cure for mononucleosis, treatment is aimed at relieving symptoms and rebuilding health. Bed rest for one to four weeks is essential to ensure a full recovery. If strep throat accompanies the mono, an antibiotic such as Erythromycin is prescribed. Drinking plenty of water flushes toxins from the system. If swallowing is difficult because of sore throat, take frequent small sips of water. Hot soups are nutritious and easier to eat than whole foods. Reduce your consumption of fats to help give your liver a rest. The liver has to work very hard to metabolize fats, and since mono affects the liver, it is important to give it time to heal. Take vitamin C for its antiviral and anti-inflammatory effects, and take vitamin E and zinc for their role in healthy immune response.

Since there is no cure for mononucleosis, treatment is aimed at relieving symptoms and rebuilding health.

Hepatitis B and C

"Hepatitis" means inflammation of the liver and can be caused by a variety of viruses. Hepatitis B has a long incubation period—usually two to four months. It is not highly contagious but can be transmitted by exposure to infected blood and by sexual contact. The virus is a very serious infection that causes jaundice, malaise, nausea, fever, rashes, itchy skin and sometimes diarrhea.

Hepatitis C has an incubation period of six weeks to six months, and its onset is marked by headache, fever, chills, weakness, vomiting, exhaustion, itching and jaundice. It usually results in an enlarged liver that is very tender. The risk factors for hepatitis C include a history of drug abuse, multiple sex partners, tattoos, and blood transfusions during surgery. If there is any doubt about the diagnosis and if liver enzymes are elevated, a hepatitis C blood test should be ordered. Even if the hepatitis C test is positive, the patient still may not have the virus, so a special PCR test needs to be done, generally by a gastroenterologist.

Treatments for hepatitis include a low-protein, low-fat diet, with multiple small meals daily. Fruits and steamed vegetables are well tolerated and nutritious. Keeping hydrated is crucial, so throughout the day sip water or diluted fruit juice, or eat fruit popsicles. During the period of acute infection, avoid acetaminophen (Tylenol) and supplements containing iron, because they are irritating to the liver. A drug that is effective against chronic hepatitis B and C is the antiviral Interferon Alfa. It can cause fatigue, but the price paid is worth it.

Lyme Disease

There are several diseases that are transmitted by the bite of an infected tick. Lyme disease is probably the most widely known, and it is a potentially long-term illness. It was first identified in Lyme, Connecticut, but it has now been found in most of the United States. Because it is spread mainly by the deer tick, the highest incidence is in places with large deer populations. However, jackrabbits and field mice also have been found to carry infected ticks.

Ticks are tiny and their bites are usually painless, so overlooking a tick bite is common. And since the symptoms of Lyme disease mimic other ailments, an early diagnosis may be missed.

The first sign will generally be a bull's eye mark at the location of the bite—ordinarily on the arm or leg. The spot then expands and is pale in the center. The bullet spot, or rash, usually is accompanied by flulike symptoms including fever, headache, achiness and fatigue. These symptoms can occur anywhere from three days to three weeks after the bite. Recovery

All patients do not experience the classic textbook symptoms of Lyme disease.

varies among individuals. Some people get better quickly, and others develop long-term complications including arthritis and neurological problems. Typically, the fatigue and achiness last for weeks; but if the body is unable to eradicate this insidious spirochete, these symptoms can last a lifetime. This is why most textbooks recommend testing for Lyme in anyone with chronic fatigue. This organism has the ability to hide in body tissues (including the brain) and break out into fresh infections periodically. Most Lyme patients have candidal intestinal overgrowth (see chapter 6).

I have seen a large number of CFS and FMS patients who have subtle Lyme disease and, upon being treated, improve. Lyme experts say one-third of patients do not remember being bitten by a tick, nor do they necessarily have the typical bullet rash. All patients do not experience the classic textbook symptoms, but it has been shown by SPECT scans that almost every chronic Lyme patient has central nervous system involvement. Although this disease is best treated early, soon after the tick bite, it can be successfully—but with more difficulty—cured later in the course of the illness. Therefore, if after spending any time outdoors you notice a bull's-eye bite or experience unexplained flulike symptoms, consult your physician. Diagnosis is made by a specific lab test—the Western Blot and/or PCA—for the Lyme bacteria. Lyme experts say that the ELISA lab test is not very accurate. Generally, tickborne diseases are curable with oral antibiotics such as Tetracycline and Doxycycline. These antibiotics should be taken for anywhere from 10 days to a month, depending on the severity of symptoms and the length of time the infection has been present, but a patient may need up to eight months of IV antibiotics.

To prevent Lyme disease, always wear a long-sleeved shirt, long pants and a hat when spending time in any area where ticks are likely to be present. Tuck your leg pants into your socks to prevent ticks from climbing up from the ground to find exposed skin. After being outdoors, thoroughly check your clothing and body for ticks, and shower as soon as possible. If you find a tick on your body, remove it with tweezers, grabbing the tick as close to your skin as possible and pulling firmly.[3] Remember that this may be the most important infection of chronic fatigue syndromes.

POLYMYALGIA RHEUMATICA OF THE ELDERLY

Polymyalgia rheumatica (PMR) is a subtle cause of fatigue in the elderly and typically also produces leg and shoulder discomfort. This illness is due to inflammation in the various blood vessels of the body and is usually occult. An ESR, or sedimentation rate, is almost always elevated. The simple treatment for this it to give cortisone in low doses for approximately four to six months. One form of polymyalgia is called temporal arteritis; it induces headaches and tenderness in the temporal region of the skull. This needs to be aggressively treated with larger does of cortisone because it can lead to blindness.

CHAPTER 9

ENDOCRINE FATIGUE

Menopause (Female and Male) and Polycystic Ovaries

The endocrine system is composed of hormone-producing glands throughout the body. The ovaries in women produce estrogen, progesterone and testosterone; and testicles in men produce testosterone. These hormones play a vital role in an individual's energy level. Menopause (both female and male) and polycystic ovaries are some conditions that can cause one to be especially susceptible to hormone-related fatigue.

FEMALE MENOPAUSE

Menopause occurs in women when their ovaries stop producing significant amounts of estrogen and menstruation ceases. This process happens gradually and generally starts when a woman is between the ages of 42 and 55. Menopause is a natural part of life, but it can cause a variety of unpleasant symptoms. Previously, I described declining estrogen levels as putting women at risk for developing chronic fatigue syndromes. We know that estrogen offers neuroprotection as well as neurotropism to the central nervous system.[1] (A neurotrophic effect implies a healthful tendency toward growth and maturation versus one that tends toward cell death.) The neuroprotective effect involves several mechanisms that improve brain metabolism, cerebral blood flow and oxidant injury.[2] It is also known that estrogen increases nitrous oxide in the vessels of the brain, which contributes to vascular health.[3] The brain chemicals acetylcholine and serotonin, which are vital for homeostasis of the brain and body, are increased by estrogen stimulation.[4] Cognitive function, sleep and energy mechanisms of the brain are just a few of the bodily actions modified by this very important female hormone. Estrogen also helps protect the brain from the effects of the stress hormone cortisol, which is secreted by the adrenal glands. With lowered levels of estrogen comes accelerated bone loss, which may put one at risk for osteoporosis.

Symptoms of low estrogen include:

- Hot flashes
- Night sweats
- Decreased vaginal lubrication
- Mood changes that tend toward depression and anxiety
- Fatigue and an emotional sense of a lack of well-being
- Headaches

It is understandable how menopause and low estrogen levels can play an important role in a woman's sense of well-being. However, as long as there is sufficient estrogen to produce a menstrual cycle, it is highly unlikely that estrogen is a major contributing factor in a fatigue-related syndrome. However, if a woman has had a total hysterectomy (surgical removal of uterus and ovaries) and has not had replacement estrogen, then fatigue could result.

Diagnosis and Treatment

Laboratory diagnosis of estrogen deficiency is fairly straightforward. If the sera FSH and LH are elevated, then estrogen is low the majority of the time. If estrogen is found to be low, then replacement hormones may be prescribed. Some physicians recommend Premarin, an oral estrogen derived from the urine of pregnant horses. Other physicians believe that estradiol-type hormones found in patches, pills or shots may be best because the only type of female estrogen receptors in the brain are estradiol receptors. Still other physicians believe that natural estrogen in the exact estradiol:estriol:estrone ratio found in a woman's body is best. The more natural forms of hormones can be obtained from a compounding pharmacist. These pharmacists actually mix the prescribed ingredients instead of dispensing premanufactured pills.

If a woman has a uterus, she needs to supplement progesterone in addition to estrogen because unopposed estrogen may induce cancers of the uterus. Natural progesterone—available in a cream from a compounding pharmacy—is preferable. There is a growing belief among physicians that natural progesterone plus estrogen may improve women's health and, in some cases, can help in fibromyalgia. However, hormone replacement therapy is not suitable for all women. If you have a history of liver disease, breast or endometrial cancer, or blood-clotting problems, it is not advisable to take estrogen. In 2002, research studies conducted with women taking the hormone Prempro (estrogen and progestogen) showed an associated risk of increased health problems. Make sure to discuss with your physician the specific advantages and risks regarding hormone replacement therapy.

Every woman's body and health history are unique, and no one therapy is appropriate for all women.

Nondrug treatments of menopausal symptoms include increasing your intake of foods containing phytoestrogens (plant estrogens). Soy products, apples, beets, barley, cabbage, oats, flaxseeds, olives, olive oil, papaya, kidney beans, rice, split peas, sunflower seeds and yams all contain substantial amounts of phytoestrogens. Avoid the foods that worsen symptoms—refined sugars, red meat, chocolate, alcohol and caffeine. Since hot flashes can contribute to dehydration, drinking six to eight glasses of pure water is essential. Exercise is important for maintaining strong muscles, preventing osteoporosis and heart disease, and improving mood. Weight-bearing exercises such as walking and running increase bone density. It is recommended that you exercise at least 30 minutes three times a week to provide lasting benefits.

Nondrug treatments of menopausal symptoms include increasing your intake of foods containing phytoestrogens (plant estrogens).

MALE MENOPAUSE

Menopause is a condition most often associated with women; however, it affects men as well. Male menopause (or andropause) is a distinct physiological phenomenon that is caused by a decrease in production of the main male hormone (or androgen) testosterone. It usually starts to occur between the ages of 45 and 60. Men can continue to father children, but their level of testosterone diminishes gradually as they age. Symptoms are generally most noticeable starting at around age 60. Male menopause does not affect all men, and the intensity of symptoms is generally less than in women.

The symptoms for low testosterone include:

- Erectile dysfunction
- Depression
- Decreased sex drive
- Lethargy
- Loss of muscle mass and muscle strength
- Low sperm count
- A reduction in bone density

Factors that contribute to the severity of the symptoms are excessive alcohol consumption, obesity, smoking, hypertension, certain medications, poor diet, lack of exercise and psychological problems such as midlife depression. An increase in circulating levels of estrogen—perhaps from ingesting hormone-treated animal products—can reduce the availability of testosterone in cells.

Treatment

The treatment for male menopause is replacement of testosterone, which can restore sexual dysfunction and reverse depression and fatigue. Testosterone is available in many forms—oral, injectable and transdermal. Because of the risk of liver toxicity, oral forms are not recommended. The newer gels, creams and patches seem to be safer and more efficient. Exercise and diet play an important role in testosterone production at any age. A protein-rich diet and strengthening activities such as weight training have been proven to be beneficial. If the symptoms of male menopause are pronounced and fatigue is troublesome, see a primary-care physician or a urologist who can do the appropriate testing and provide the appropriate treatment.

POLYCYSTIC OVARIES

A significant cause of fatigue in young- to middle-aged women is a condition called polycystic ovaries (PCO), which is a hormonal malfunction. It occurs when a woman's ovaries produce too many androgens, or male hormones. Testosterone is the main androgen.

The following are the usual characteristics of PCO:

- Increased hair on the chin, upper lip, abdomen or upper chest
- Acne
- Menstrual irregularities
- A history of ovarian cysts
- Increased masculinity with deepening of voice and possible hair loss
- A history of infertility or difficulty in becoming pregnant
- A tendency toward diabetes
- Obesity
- Fatigue and lethargy

Origin

There is no proven cause of PCO. This condition is hereditary in some cases, but most cases are not genetic in origin. Because chronic testosterone overproduction blocks the normal growth and development of eggs in the ovaries, the ovaries contain many small cysts from underdeveloped eggs, which show up on an ultrasound—hence the name polycystic ovaries. There is an association between obesity and PCO. About 50 percent of women with this condition have excess body fat. Half of the cases of hirsutism (excessive body hair) are actually due to PCO. Insulin resistance, which is defined as resistance of the body to the action of insulin absorbing glucose from the bloodstream into the cells, is common in PCO. Therefore, a tendency toward diabetes can occur. Glucose-tolerance test results are usually abnormal in patients with PCO. The psychological aspects of this syndrome also can be devastating, since infertility, body hair, obesity and fatigue are side effects. Therefore, depression is often associated with PCO.

Diagnosis and Treatment

An elevated testosterone level can substantiate a PCO diagnosis. If this is discovered, additional definitive tests need to be done to rule out other testosterone-producing illnesses such as tumors, genetic problems and certain enzyme defects from childhood. An LH to FSH ratio (pituitary hormones) greater than two is very common in PCO and should give the clinician cause for suspicion.

Once recognized, the treatment of this syndrome is fairly straightforward. Many physicians prescribe Glucophage or one of the troglitazones (Avandia or Actos) to decrease insulin resistance. This dramatically helps fatigue, decreases the body hair and reverses many of the other problems associated with the condition. The use of a 2 percent progesterone cream can help alleviate symptoms in some women. The fatigue is almost completely reversible with treatment. Other treatments also are available, but the patient should see an endocrinologist.

Case Report

A 28-year-old infertile young woman seeking spiritual counseling came to my office. We discussed certain emotional problems she was having (mainly unresolved anger and several rejection experiences), but I began to suspect from her symptoms of hirsutism, obesity, fatigue and sugar craving that she might have PCO. Her testosterone levels were elevated and other rarer syndromes were ruled out, so I began her on Glucophage. Within weeks, she felt dramatically better and was extremely happy with the diagnosis and treatment, especially because previous visits to OB/GYN doctors had failed to diagnose her correctly.

CHAPTER 10

FOR PHYSICIANS:
A SYSTEMATIC
APPROACH TO
DIAGNOSIS AND
TREATMENT

It is good for thee to dwell deep, that thou mayest feel and understand the spirits of people.

JOHN WOOLMAN

Since the symptom of fatigue itself can have thousands of etiologies and virtually every disease or syndrome can cause this symptom, one would think it would be very difficult to find the cause and treat it. However, that is not necessarily the case if one uses a systematic approach. If after the typical lab tests and

X rays are done you still don't have an answer, keep in mind the four major fatigue syndromes discussed in chapter 3-6 and the others mentioned in chapters 7-9. The underlying criterion for finding the cause of fatigue is to listen to and *believe the patient*.

Ninety percent of diagnoses will be found within the patient's history. If you listen to the patient long enough, they will tell you what's wrong with them.

As we all learned in medical school, 90 percent of diagnoses will be found within the patient's history. If you listen to the patient long enough, they will tell you what's wrong with them. It may mean spending extra time in consultation, but what you learn can be more valuable than test results. The remaining 10 percent of diagnoses are discovered with lab and X-ray results and a physical exam. When talking with a patient, I focus on the patient's history and symptoms:

1. Exactly what does the patient mean by fatigue? Does the patient mean his or her muscles tire out? Feel sleepy? Have brain fog? Is there a sense of heaviness in the arms and legs? Sometimes a person will say, "I am tired from my waist down." Does the patient have claudication? Is he or she tired at rest?

2. The onset of the symptom is extremely important. Was there a sudden onset? Has it been gradual? What has been the duration? Does it worsen during certain times of the year? In response to changes in weather? In response to exposure to certain chemicals or to ingestion of certain foods?

3. Is pain associated with the fatigue? If the patient has pain and tender muscles, then the obvious syndrome

to rule out is fibromyalgia. This is probably the easiest of the four syndromes to diagnose. Other syndromes that cause pain include chronic fatigue syndrome, depression and polymyalgia rheumatica of the elderly. Sometimes severe perennial allergies will induce aching. Other painful conditions are obvious, such as arthritis, migraine headaches and the like.

4. Does the patient experience fever or night sweats and sore throat? If so, think of chronic fatigue syndrome, allergies or chronic sinusitis, among others. You must always rule out lymphoma.

5. Prior to the onset of fatigue, was the patient given antibiotics? Is he or she taking hormones? Has he or she had major surgery? Been in a car accident? Had a neck or back injury? Does he or she spend eight hours a day sitting at a computer?

6. Does the patient experience coldness, hair loss, weight gain and constipation, depression and sluggishness? If yes, then you should consider hypothyroidism or some other endocrine disorder.

7. Does the patient experience multisystem symptoms? If yes, then suggest neurotoxic type diseases. In addition, a FACT test should be ordered.

8. Chemical and toxic history should be obtained. Does the patient live in an agricultural community where insecticides are sprayed or in an industrial area? His or her work environment should be discussed. Sometimes a heavy metal screen that is provoked by DMSO may be important.

9. What are the patient's sleep habits? Does he or she have sleep onset difficulties? Snore? Wake up in the middle of the night and can't return to sleep? Feel rested after a night's sleep?

10. Does the patient have a family history of any psychiatric disorders such as bipolar illness, depression or anxiety? Has there been a life stress event? Does the patient have crying spells, loss of interest in life or a loss of pleasure?

11. Ask about the patient's dietary history. Does he or she smoke, drink alcohol or take illicit drugs? Drink a lot of caffeine or eat MSG? Drink diet sodas containing NutraSweet? Does the patient crave or eat any particular food—especially sugars, simple starches and junk foods? Does he or she crave salty foods? How much water does he or she drink?

12. Are there emotional or spiritual problems that are evident? Is there an unhealthy lifestyle contrary to the principles of Scripture? Is the patient overwhelmed by ongoing mental or physical stresses?

In addition to this, a thorough review of other specific factors can help expose the source of illness. I always ask, for example, if there is a history of travel or tick bites or possible exposure to malaria. (Note: I have diagnosed five patients with recurring malaria, which had been overlooked by other physicians and specialists. Appropriate treatment resulted in complete remission.)

A tier of suggested testing can be found in chapter 3. My overriding clinical concern is always that of an occult malignancy or some type of connective tissue disease, so I always ask about night sweats, fevers and weight loss. If the patient does have these symptoms and one is unsure of the diagnosis, a CT scan of the chest and abdomen are in order. Dull abdominal pain may be a clue to early lymphoma, carcinoma of the kidney or pancreatic cancer. Dull abdominal pain with constipation or diarrhea may also indicate yeast overgrowth.

CASE HISTORY

A middle-aged farmer with a history of a viral-type infection recently came to my office. He suffered from fatigue, fever and night sweats. His sedimentation rate was in the 80s and 90s. My first concern was that of an occult malignancy. After additional lab tests were basically within normal limits and a chest X ray showed very little, I ordered a CT scan of the chest and abdomen. To my surprise, the CT showed pericarditis, which was not clearly seen on the chest X ray. I referred him to a local cardiologist, and after appropriate doses of prednisone, the patient eventually returned to his usual health.

TESTS

Basic lab tests include CBC, ESR, uric acid, comprehensive metabolic profile, ANA, RA, T7, TSH, KOH or wet prep of the mouth, urinalysis, serum B12 and folate. Other lab and X-ray tests include a chest X ray, HIV antibody, hepatitis B and C screen, PPD, HAM-D or MMPI, Lyme serology, Brucella titers, HHV-6 antibodies, Parvovirus, IGM, CMV, Epstein-Barr titer, Monospot, CNS of nares, transesophageal echocardiogram, fungal antibodies, Tensilon test, 24-hour urine keto- and hydroxysteroids, ACTH test and, as stated above, a DMSO provocation for heavy metals. (Note: Many environmental specialists do not consider a 24-hour urine and/or hair analysis for heavy metals a reliable standard.) Any chronic allergy sufferer needs to have a sinus X ray or CT scan of the sinuses. Other lab and X-ray modalities may need to be ordered based on the patient's symptoms.

CONCLUSION

In closing, I do not improve or resolve fatigue in every patient. There are some that are just enigmatic. However, if the patient perceives that you are caring and supportive, he or she will be more likely to respond to your treatment. If you are willing to refer patients to other physicians—traditional or nontradition-al—the patient will know that you are more concerned with his or her well-being than your own need to be infallible. Even if you refer patients to a medical school or teaching university and a definitive diagnosis still cannot be made, continue to investigate and keep an open mind. Patients who returned to my clinic after having been to numerous specialists have stated that I've helped them more than these experts. I think they respond to the compassionate, personal approach given by our office.

CLINICAL LOGIC

If an illness or syndrome is widespread and debilitating,
search for a cure.
If an answer is unproven but appears logical,
pursue it.
If the treatment is benign,
try it.
If it doesn't work,
nothing lost.
If it does work,
great gain.
But it may be a placebo effect.
So what?
But the placebo may modify an unknown pathologic mechanism.
A discovery.
But the smart guys and the critics won't accept it.
Who cares?
If you try such treatment and it works, your patient will thank you. He or she could not care less about your unbelieving colleagues.
He or she is well.

If you are a doctor, don't give up. If you are a patient, don't give up. Incredible discoveries are being made in medicine, and new naturopathic treatments are being proven effective. Because we have a powerful sovereign God who cares about us, we should keep looking and listening and never give up hope. He will provide wisdom and healing to those who seek Him.

The Sovereign LORD has given me an instructed tongue, to know the word that sustains the weary. *He wakens me morning by morning, wakens my ear to listen like one being taught. The Sovereign LORD has opened my ears.*

ISAIAH 50:4, EMPHASIS ADDED

RESOURCES

Dr. Jonathan Forester's Website

www.DoctorForester.com

ORGANIZATIONS

Centers for Disease Control and Prevention
1600 Clifton Road
Atlanta, GA 30333
www.cdc.gov

Christian Oasis (Dr. Forester's retreat center)
2803 Donahue Ferry
Pineville, LA 71360

HealthWatch Newsletter (CFS and FMS information)
Pro Health
2040 Alameda Padre Serra, Suite 101
Santa Barbara, CA 93103
(800) 366-6056
www.immunesupport.com/healthwatch

Lyme Disease Network
www.LymeNet.org

National Institutes of Health
9000 Rockville Pike
Bethesda, MD 20892
www.nih.gov

Share, Care and Prayer
P.O. Box 2080
Frazier Park, CA 93225
www.sharecareprayer.org

Visual Contrast Sensitivity Test Center
500 Market Street
Pocomoke City, MD 21851
www.chronicneurotoxins.com

ENDNOTES

Chapter 2

1. R. E. Morrison and H. J. Keating, III, "Fatigue in Primary Care," *Obstetrics and Gynecology Clinics of America,* vol. 28, no. 2 (June 2001), pp. 225-240.
2. G. G. May, *Addiction and Grace* (San Francisco, CA: Harper San Francisco, 1988), pp. 69-72.
3. Ibid.
4. S. Wessely, "Chronic Fatigue: Symptom and Syndrome," *Annals of Internal Medicine,* vol. 134, no. 9 (May 2001), pp. 838-843.

Chapter 3

1. List provided by the Centers for Disease Control and Prevention.
2. For more information, see the Centers for Disease Control and Prevention website at http://www.cdc.gov/ncidod/diseases/cfs.
3. G. Cowley, M. Hagar and N. Joseph, "Chronic Fatigue Syndrome," *Newsweek,* vol. 11/12 (1990), pp. 67-70.
4. G. P. Holmes et al., "Chronic Fatigue Syndrome: A Working Case Definition," *Annals of Internal Medicine,* vol. 108 (1988), pp. 387-389.
5. B. H. Natelson et al., "Is Depression Associated with Immune Activation?" *Journal of Affective Disorders,* vol. 53 (1999), pp. 179-184.
6. Ibid.
7. Ibid.
8. G. Krueger et al., "Dynamics of Chronic Active Herpesvirus-6 Infection in Patients with Chronic Fatigue Syndrome: Data Acquisition for Computer modeling," *In Vivo,* vol. 15, no. 6 (November-December 2001), pp. 461-462.
9. G. L. Nicholson et al., "Chronic Infections as a Common Etiology for Many Patients with Chronic Fatigue Syndrome, Fibromyalgia and Gulf War Illness," *Journal of Internal Medicine,* vol. 1 (1998), pp. 42-46.
10. C. G. Fisher, *Chronic Fatigue Syndrome* (New York: Warner Books, 1977), pp. 67-68.
11. V. Carpanan, "CFIDS Treatment: The Cheney Clinic's Strategic Approach," *The CFIDS Chronicle* (spring 1995), pp. 38-45.
12. Christy Weir, personal letter to several doctors in her community, 2001.
13. S. Milana et al., "Intraperitoneal Injection of Tetracyclines Protects Mice from Lethal Endotoxemia-Down-Regulating Inducible Nitric Oxide

Synthase in Various Organs and Cytokine and Nitrate Secretion in Blood," *Antimicrobial Agents Chemotherapy*, vol. 41, no. 1 (January 1997), pp. 117-121.

14. For more information, see the Visual Contrast Sensitivity Test Center's website at http://www.chronicneurotoxins.com.

15. R. C. Shoemaker, *Desperation Medicine* (Baltimore, MD: Gateway Press, 2001), pp. 457-458.

Chapter 4

1. Since FMS and CFS are very similar, fibromyalgia sufferers should read chapter 3 on chronic fatigue syndrome as well.

2. This testimony is from one of Dr. Forester's FMS patients. The names of his patients have not been included for the privacy of these individuals.

3. D. Clauw et al, "Fibromyalgia: Diagnosis and Management," *American Family Physician*, vol. 62, no. 7 (Oct. 2000), pp. 1575-1582.

4. This testimony is from one of Dr. Forester's FMS patients. The names of his patients have not been included for the privacy of these individuals.

5. S. R. Pillemer et al., "The Neuroscience and Endocrinology of Fibromyalgia," *Arthritis and Rheumatology*, vol. 40 (1997), pp. 1928-1939.

6. D. L. Goldenberg, "Fibromyalgia Syndrome a Decade Later: What Have We Learned?" *Archives of Internal Medicine*, vol. 159 (1999), pp. 777-785

7. For more information, see the National Institutes of Health website at http://www.nih.gov.

8. I. J. Russell, II, M.D., et al., "Elevated Cerebrospinal Fluid Levels of Substance P in Patients with the Fibromyalgia Syndrome," *Arthritis and Rheumatology*, vol. 31 (1994), pp. 1593-1601.

9. P. A. Weigent, J. E. Bradley and G. S. Allarron, "Current Concepts in the Pathophysiology of Abnormal Pain Perception in Fibromyalgia," *American Journal of Medical Science*, vol. 315 (1998), pp. 405-412.

10. H. Cohen et al., "Autonomic Nervous System Derangement in Fibromyalgia Syndrome and Related Disorders," *The Israel Medical Association Journal*, vol. 10 (October 3, 2001), pp. 755-760.

11. D. J. Wallace and J. B. Wallace, *Making Sense of Fibromyalgia* (New York: Oxford University Press, 1999), pp. 113-118.

12. V. Carpanan, "CFIDS Treatment: The Cheney Clinic's Strategic Approach," The CFIDS Chronicle (spring 1995), pp. 38-45.

13. This list of secondary symptoms is provided by Patricia Drexler, an FMS patient.

14. *Neuroplasticity*. "An Introduction and Implications for Therapy." http://www.sohp.soton.ac.uk/neuro/pres/plasti.ppt (accessed May 21, 2003).

15. E. A. Newsholme, P. Calder and P. Yaqoob, "The Regulating, Informational,

and Immunomodulatory Roles of Fat Fuels," American Journal of Nutrition, vol. 57, suppl. 5 (1993), pp. 738S-750S.

16. M. M. Dwight et al., "An Open Clinical Trial of Venlafaxine Treatment of Fibromyalgia," Psychosomatics vol. 39 (1998), pp. 14-17.

Chapter 5

1. Michael T. McDermot, *Endocrine Secrets,* 3rd ed. (Philadelphia: Handley and Belfus, 2002), pp. 306-307.

2. Gorman B. McIver, "Euthyroid Sick Syndrome: An Overview," *Thyroid,* vol. 7 (1997), pp. 125-132.

3. L. M. Demers and C. A. Spencer, eds. "Laboratory Medicine Practice Guidelines: Laboratory Support for the Diagnosis and Monitoring of Thyroid Disease," *National Academy of Clinical Biochemistry,* January 20, 2001. http://www.nacb.org/lmpg/thyroid_lmpg.stm (accessed January 2002).

4. Richard L. Shames, M.D. and Karilee H. Shames, *Thyroid Power* (New York: HarperCollins Publishers, 2002), p. 79.

5. Ridha Arem, M.D., *The Thyroid Solution* (New York: Ballantine Books, 2000), pp. 223-230.

6. J. C. Lowe and G. Honeyman-Lowe, "Fibromyalgia and Thyroid Disease" (proceedings of the conference of the French Fibromyalgia Association, Grenoble, France, May, 1999).

7. Shames and Shames, *Thyroid Power*, pp. 223-230.

Chapter 6

1. For more information, see the *The Candida Page*, a list of websites about *Candida albicans* and candidiasis, at http://www.candidapage.com.

2. Gerald L. Mandell, John E. Bennett and Raphael Dolin, eds., "Infectious Diseases and their Etiologic Agents," *Principles and Practice of Infectious Disease*, vol. 2 (2000), pp. 2656-2657.

3. W. G. Crook, *The Yeast Connection* (New York: Vintage Books, 1986).

4. For more information, see *The Chronic Candidiasis Syndrome* website at http://www.cfs-recovery.org/docdarren2.html.

5. Jann Weiss, "The Candida/Aldehyde Detox Pathway and the Molybdenum Connection," *The Candida Page*, January 2, 2002. http://www.candida-page.com/aldehyde.shtml (accessed January 2002).

6. W. G. Crook, *The Yeast Connection and the Woman* (Jackson, TN: Professional Books, 1998), p. 86.

7. C. P. Jessop, report of work with 11,000 patients (report presented at the Chronic Fatigue Syndrome Conference, San Francisco, CA, April 15, 1989).

8. W. G. Crook, *Tired—So Tired! and the Yeast Connection* (Jackson, TN: Professional Books, 2001), pp. 167-171.

9. J. A. Como and W. E. Dismukes, "Oral Azo-drugs as Systemic Anti-Fungal Therapy," *New England Journal of Medicine,* vol. 330 (1994), pp. 263-272.

10. W. G. Crook, *A Special Message to the Health Professional* (Jackson, TN: International Health Foundation, Inc., 1998), n.p.

11. Ibid.

12. R. E. Cater, II, M.D., "Chronic Intestinal Candidiasis as a Possible Etiologic Factor in Chronic Fatigue Syndrome," *Medical Hypothesis,* vol. 44 (1995), pp. 507-515.

Chapter 7

1. A. Chaudhuri and P. O. Behan, "Fatigue and Basal Ganglia," *Journal of Neurological Sciences,* vol. 179 (2000), pp. 34-42.

2. S. M. Stahl, "The Psychopharmacology of Energy and Fatigue," *Journal of Clinical Psychiatry,* vol. 63, no. 1 (2002), pp. 7-8.

3. F. Minirth, *Love Hunger: Recovery from Food Addiction* (New York: Fawcett Book Group, 1991), pp. 12-13.

Chapter 8

1. *Medical Letter,* vol. 44, p. 1126.

2. G. H. Ross et al., "Neurotoxicity in Single Proton Emission Compared Tomography Brain Scans of Patients Reporting Chemical Sensitivities," *Toxicology and Industrial Health,* vol. 15 (1999), pp. 414-420.

3. For more information about Lyme disease, visit www.LymeNet.org.

Chapter 9

1. D. O. Murphy and M. Segal, "Regulation of Dendritic Spine Density in Cultured Hippocanthal Neurons by Steroid Hormones," *The Journal of Neuroscience: The Official Journal of the Society for Neuroscience,* vol. 16, no. 13 (1996), pp. 4059-4068.

2. W. Rudzinski and J. Krejza, "Effects of Estrogens on the Brain and Implications for Neuroprotection," *Neurologia Neurochirurgia Polska,* vol. 36, no. 1 (January/February 2002), pp. 143-156.

3. A. McNeill et. al., "Estrogen Increases Endothelial Nitric Oxide Synthase via Estrogen Receptors in Rat Cerebral Blood Vessels: Effect Preserved After Concurrent Treatment with Medroxyprogesterone Acetate or Progesterone," *Stroke,* vol. 33, no. 6 (June 2002), pp. 685-691.

4. Rudzinski and Krejza, "Effects of Estrogens on the Brain," pp. 143-156.

GLOSSARY

acetaldehyde—A colorless volatile water-soluble liquid aldehyde that can cause irritation to mucous membranes.

acidophilus—Species of bacteria (*Lactobacillus acidophilus*) that is normally found in a healthy intestine.

ACTH—A protein hormone of the anterior lobe of the pituitary gland that stimulates the adrenal cortex. Also called adreno-corticotropic hormone.

adrenal gland—One of two glands located above the kidneys that secrete a number of key hormones including epinephrine and cortisol.

AIDS—A disease of the human immune system that is characterized by a reduction in the number of helper T cells to 20 percent or less of normal, thereby rendering the subject highly vulnerable to life-threatening conditions (such as Pneumocystis carinii pneumonia) and to some conditions that can become life-threatening (such as Kaposi's sarcoma), and that is caused by infection with HIV commonly transmitted in infected blood, especially during intravenous drug use and in bodily secretions (such as semen) during sexual intercourse. Also called acquired immune deficiency syndrome or acquired immunodeficiency syndrome.

alpha wave—An electrical rhythm of the brain with a frequency of 8 to 13 cycles per second that is often associated with a state of wakeful relaxation.

anabolic steroid—Any of a group of usually synthetic hormones that increase constructive metabolism and are sometimes abused by athletes to increase temporarily the size of their muscles.

anaphylactic shock—An often severe and sometimes fatal systemic reaction in a susceptible individual upon a second exposure to a specific antigen (such as wasp venom or penicillin) after previous sensitization that is characterized especially by respiratory symptoms, fainting, itching and hives.

anaphylaxis—Hypersensitivity (as to foreign proteins or drugs) resulting from sensitization following prior contact with the causative agent.

androgen—A male sex hormone (such as testosterone).

anhedonia—A psychological condition characterized by the inability to experience pleasure in acts which normally produce it.

antibody—Protein created by the immune system in response to the presence of a foreign organism or toxin that is capable of destroying or neutralizing the invader. Also called immunoglobulin.

antigen—A substance (such as a toxin or enzyme) capable of stimulating an immune response.

antimicrobial—Destroying or inhibiting the growth of microorganisms, or an agent that is capable of doing this.

antioxidant—Substance that blocks oxidation reactions in the body, some of which can lead to cellular dysfunction and destruction.

anxiolytic—A drug that relieves anxiety.

arthralgia—Pain in one or more joints.

autoimmune disorder—Condition in which the immune system attacks the body's own tissue and interferes with normal functioning.

autonomic nervous system—A part of the nervous system that innervates smooth and cardiac muscle and glandular tissues and governs involuntary actions (such as secretion, vasoconstriction or peristalsis) and that consists of the sympathetic nervous system and the parasympathetic nervous system.

autonomic—Acting or occurring involuntarily; relating to, affecting or controlled by the autonomic nervous system.

benzodiazepine—Any of a group of aromatic lipophilic amines (such as diazepam and chlordiazepoxide) used especially as tranquilizers.

bipolar disorder—Any of several mood disorders characterized usually by alternating episodes of depression and mania. Also called bipolar affective disorder, bipolar illness, manic depression, manic-depressive psychosis.

candida—A genus of parasitic fungi of the order Moniliales that resemble yeasts; occur especially in the mouth, vagina and intestinal tract; are usually benign but can become pathogenic; and include the causative agent of thrush (*C. albicans*).

candidiasis—Infection with or disease caused by a fungus of the genus *Candida*.

CAT scan—Computerized axial tomography scan; a diagnostic test that uses computers and X rays to construct a three-dimensional picture of the body's structures and organs. Also called CT scan.

CFS—*See* **chronic fatigue syndrome.**

chronic fatigue syndrome—A disorder of uncertain cause that is characterized by persistent profound fatigue usually accompanied by impairment in short-term memory or concentration, sore throat, tender lymph nodes, muscle or joint pain and headache unrelated to any preexisting medical condition, and that typically has an onset at about 30 years of age. Abbreviated CFS. Also called myalgic encephalomyelitis or chronic fatigue immune deficiency syndrome.

CNS—Central nervous system.

corticosteroid—Steroid hormone produced by the adrenal gland, or a synthetic version of such a hormone.

corticotropin-releasing factor—A substance secreted by the hypothalamus that regulates the release of ACTH by the anterior lobe of the pituitary gland. Abbreviated CRF.

cortisol—*See* **hydrocortisone.**

CRF—*See* **corticotropin-releasing factor.**

CPAP—Continuous positive airway pressure.

cytokine—Any of a class of immunoregulatory proteins (such as interleukin, tumor necrosis factor, and interferon) that are secreted by cells especially of the immune system.

DA—*See* **dopamine.**

dehydroepiandrosterone—An androgenic steroid secreted by the adrenal cortex that is an intermediate in the biosynthesis of testosterone. Abbreviated DHA or DHEA.

delta wave—A high-amplitude electrical rhythm of the brain with a frequency of less than 6 hertz that occurs especially in deep sleep, in infancy and in many diseased conditions of the brain.

DHA—*See* **dehydroepiandrosterne.**

DHEA—*See* **dehydroepiandrosterone.**

dopamine—A monoamine that is a form of dopa and occurs especially as a neurotransmitter in the brain and as an intermediate in the biosynthesis of epinephrine. Abbreviated DA.

dysautonomia—A disorder of the autonomic nervous system that causes disturbances in all or some autonomic functions and may result from the course of a disease (such as diabetes) or from injury or poisoning.

dysthymia—A mood disorder characterized by chronic mildly depressed or irritable mood often accompanied by other symptoms (such as eating and sleeping disturbances, fatigue and poor self-esteem).

EBV—*See* **Epstein-Barr virus.**

EFA—*See* **essential fatty acid.**

ELISA test—Enzyme-linked immunoadsorbent assay; test that determines the presence of a particular protein (such as an antibody) in the blood or other body fluid.

encephalopathy—A disease of the brain, especially one involving alterations of brain structure.

endocrine system—The glands and parts of glands that secrete hormones into the bloodstream to help integrate and control metabolic activity; these include the pituitary, thyroid, parathyroids, adrenals, pancreas, ovaries and testes.

endorphin—Any of a number of hormonelike substances found especially in the brain; one function being to suppress the sensation of pain by binding to receptors in the brain (a function imitated by narcotic drugs).

epinephrine—A hormone that is the principal blood-pressure-raising hormone secreted by the adrenal medulla, is prepared from adrenal extracts or made synthetically, and is used medicinally especially as a heart stimulant, as a vasoconstrictor in controlling hemorrhages of the skin and in prolonging the effects of local anesthetics, and as a muscle relaxant in bronchial asthma. Also called adrenaline.

Epstein-Barr virus—A herpesvirus (genus *Lymphocryptovirus*) that causes infectious mononucleosis and is associated with Burkitt's lymphoma and nasopharyngeal carcinoma. Abbreviated EBV. Also called EB virus.

essential fatty acid—Any of the many organic acids of which fats and oils are composed that the body requires but cannot manufacture on its own and that therefore must be supplied through the diet. Abbreviated EFA.

estradiol—A natural hormone that is secreted chiefly by the ovaries, is the most potent of the naturally occurring estrogens and is administered in its natural or semisynthetic esterified form, especially to treat menopausal symptoms.

etiology—The cause or causes of a disease or abnormal condition.

euthyroid—Characterized by normal thyroid function.

fibromyalgia—Functional disorder that causes pain in the muscles, joints, ligaments and tendons, with distinct points on the body that are tender to the touch; characterized by increased sensitivity to pain, sleep difficulties and fatigue. Abbreviated FMS. Also called fibromyositis.

FMS—*See* **fibromyalgia.**

follicle-stimulating hormone—A hormone from an anterior lobe of the pituitary gland that stimulates the growth of the ovum-containing follicles in the ovary and activates sperm-forming cells.

free radical—An especially reactive atom or group of atoms that has one or more unpaired electrons, especially one that is produced in the body by natural biological processes or introduced from outside (such as in tobacco smoke, toxins or pollutants) and that can damage cells, proteins and DNA by altering their chemical structure.

FSH—*See* **follicle-stimulating hormone.**

GABA—*See* **gamma-aminobutyric acid.**

gamma-aminobutyric acid—An amino acid that is a neurotransmitter that induces inhibition of postsynaptic neurons. Abbreviated GABA.

glutamic acid—An amino acid that is widely distributed in plant and animal proteins and that acts throughout the central nervous system as a neurotransmitter which excites postsynaptic neurons.

glutathione—A peptide that contains one amino acid residue each of glutamic acid, cysteine and glycine; that occurs widely in plant and animal tissues; and that plays an important role in biological oxidation-reduction processes and as a coenzyme.

HHV-6—A human herpesvirus (genus *Roseolovirus*) that causes roseola infantum and that tends to be associated with chronic fatigue syndrome but has not been established as its causative agent.

hirsutism—Excessive growth of hair of normal or abnormal distribution.

histamine—A compound especially of mammalian tissues that causes dilatation of capillaries, contraction of smooth muscle and stimulation of gastric acid secretion, that is released during allergic reactions.

HIV—Any of several retroviruses and especially HIV-1 that infect and destroy helper T cells of the immune system, causing the marked reduction in their numbers that is diagnostic of AIDS. Also called AIDS virus or human immunodeficiency virus.

homeostasis—The maintenance of relatively stable internal physiological conditions (such as body temperature or the pH of blood) under fluctuating environmental conditions; also the process of maintaining a stable psychological state in the individual under varying psychological pressures.

hydrocortisone—A glucocorticoid of the adrenal cortex that is a derivative of cortisone and is used in the treatment of rheumatoid arthritis. Also called cortisol.

hydrogenation—Chemical process used to turn liquid oils into more solid form by bombarding the oil molecules with hydrogen, resulting in the formation of trans-fatty acids, which do not occur in nature and have effects in the body like those of saturated fats.

hydrotherapy—The therapeutic use of water (such as a whirlpool bath).

hypotension—Abnormally low blood pressure.

hypothyroidism—Deficient activity of the thyroid gland; also a resultant bodily condition characterized by lowered metabolic rate and general loss of vigor.

immunodeficiency—Failure of the immune system to function normally in response to disease, infection or other toxins. *See also* **AIDS.**

immunotherapy—Treatment of or prophylaxis against disease by attempting to produce active or passive immunity; administration of allergy shots. Also called immune therapy.

immune system—Organs, cells, tissues and proteins that work in a coordinated manner to fight off invaders such as viruses and harmful bacteria.

immune therapy—*See* **immunotherapy.**

insulin resistance—Reduced sensitivity to insulin by the body's insulin-dependent processes (such as glucose uptake and inhibition of glucose production by the liver) that results in lowered activity of these processes or an increase in insulin production or both and that is typical of type 2 diabetes but often occurs in the absence of diabetes.

intrinsic factor—A substance produced by the normal gastrointestinal mucosa that facilitates absorption of vitamin B12.

LH—*See* **luteinizing hormone.**

luteinizing hormone—A hormone of protein-carbohydrate composition that is obtained from the pituitary gland and that together with follicle-stimulating hormone in the female stimulates the secretion of progesterone and in the male the secretion of testosterone. Abbreviated LH.

Lyme disease—An acute inflammatory disease that is usually characterized initially by the bull's-eye shaped skin lesion erythema migrans and by fatigue, fever and chills and, if left untreated, may later manifest itself in cardiac and neurological disorders, joint pain and arthritis, and that is caused by a spirochete of the genus *Borrelia* (*B. burgdorferi*), which is transmitted by the bite of a tick.

lymph—Clear fluid in which all the body's cells are bathed; provides nourishment to the cells and collects waste products given off by cells.

lymphocyte—Any of the cells that originate from stem cells and are elements of lymph, that include the cellular mediators of immunity and that constitute 20 to 30 percent of the white blood cells of normal human blood. *See also* **T cell.**

MAOI—*See* **monoamine oxidase inhibitor.**

MCS—Multiple chemical sensitivity.

ME—*See* **myalgic encephalomyelitis.**

melatonin—A hormone that is derived from serotonin, is secreted by the pineal gland (especially in response to darkness) and has been linked to the regulation of sleep/wake cycles.

mitochondrion—Any of various round or long cellular organelles that are found outside the nucleus, produce energy for the cell through cellular respiration and are rich in fats, proteins and enzymes.

monoamine oxidase inhibitor—Any various antidepressant drugs that increase the concentration of monoamines in the brain by inhibiting the action of monoamine oxidase. Abbreviated MAOI.

myalgia—Pain in one or more muscles.

myalgic encephalomyelitis—*See* **chronic fatigue syndrome.** Abbreviated ME.

myofascial—Of or relating to the fasciae of muscles.

NE—*See* **norepinephrine.**

nerve growth factor—A protein that promotes development of the sensory and sympathetic nervous systems and is required for maintenance of sympathetic neurons. Abbreviated NGF.

neural—Of, relating to or affecting a nerve or the nervous system.

neurally mediated hypotension—Condition in which the body has difficulty regulating blood pressure, especially when standing upright. Abbreviated NMH.

neurochemistry—Chemical processes and phenomena related to the nervous system.

neuromodulator—Something (such as a polypeptide) that potentiates or inhibits the transmission of a nerve impulse but is not the actual means of transmission itself.

neuropathy—An abnormal and usually degenerative state of the nervous system or nerves; also a systemic condition (such as muscular atrophy) that stems from a neuropathy.

neurotransmitter—A chemical (such as norepinephrine or acetylcholine) that transmits impulses between nerve cells in the brain and nervous system.

NGF—*See* **nerve growth factor.**

NMDA—N-methyl D-aspartate; a synthetic amino acid that binds selectively to glutamate receptors on neurons where the binding of glutamate results in the opening of calcium channels.

NMH—*See* **neurally mediated hypotension.**

norepinephrine—A neurotransmitter of the sympathetic nervous system and in some parts of the central nervous system; a vasopressor hormone of the adrenal medulla, and a precursor of epinephrine. Abbreviated NE.

NSAID—A nonsteroidal anti-inflammatory drug often used as a painkiller (such as ibuprofen).

omega-3 fatty acid—An essential fatty acid found in flaxseed oil and fish oils that helps to lower blood-fat levels, enhance efficiency of the immune system and decrease inflammation.

oxidation—Chemical reaction in which oxygen reacts with another substance causing a chemical transformation, often resulting in some type of spoilage or deterioration.

parasympathetic nervous system—The part of the autonomic nervous system that tends to induce secretion, to increase the tone and contractility of smooth muscle and to slow the heart rate. Abbreviated PNS.

pathogen—A specific causative agent (such as a bacterium or virus) of disease.

pathology—The anatomic and physiological deviations from the normal that constitute disease or characterize a particular disease.

pathophysiology—The physiology of abnormal states; specifically the functional changes that accompany a particular syndrome or disease.

PCO—Polycystic ovaries.

pernicious anemia—A severe anemia marked by a progressive decrease in number and increase in size and hemoglobin content of the red blood cells and by pallor, weakness and gastrointestinal and nervous disturbances, and associated with reduced ability to absorb vitamin B12 due to the absence of intrinsic factor.

pharmacology—The properties and reactions of drugs especially with relation to their therapeutic value.

physiology—The organic processes and phenomena of an organism or any of its parts or of a particular bodily process.

phytoestrogen—A chemical compound that occurs naturally in plants and has estrogenic properties.

pituitary—Gland located at the base of the brain that secretes hormones that regulate growth and metabolism as well as coordinating the actions of other endocrine glands.

PNS—*See* **parasympathetic nervous system.**

polycystic ovary syndrome—A variable disorder that is marked especially by amenorrhea, hirsutism, obesity, infertility and ovarian enlargement and is usually initiated by an elevated level of luteinizing hormone, androgen or estrogen.

polymyalgia rheumatica—Disorder of the elderly characterized by muscular pain and stiffness in the shoulders and neck and in the pelvic area.

probiotic—Bacteria that help to establish healthy flora in the intestines; taken as supplements, probiotics can aid digestion and increase the body's resistance to infection.

progesterone—A female steroid/sex hormone that is secreted by the corpus luteum to prepare the endometrium for implantation and later by the placenta during pregnancy to prevent rejection of the developing embryo or fetus and that is used in synthetic forms as a birth control pill, to treat menstrual disorders and to alleviate some cases of infertility.

REM sleep—A state of sleep that recurs cyclically several times during a normal period of sleep and that is characterized by depressed muscle tone and by dreaming and rapid eye movements. Also called rapid eye movement sleep.

saturated fat—Type of fat characterized by its inability to incorporate additional hydrogen atoms; solid at room temperature (e.g., butter or lard); found primarily in foods of animal origin.

SE—*See* **serotonin.**

serotonin—A neurotransmitter that is a powerful vasoconstrictor and is found especially in the brain, blood serum and gastric mucous membrane. Abbreviated SE.

sleep apnea—Brief periods of recurrent cessation of breathing during sleep that is caused especially by obstruction of the airway or a disturbance in the brain's respiratory center and is associated especially with excessive daytime sleepiness.

SNS—*See* **sympathetic nervous system.**

somatic—Of, relating to or affecting the body, especially as distinguished from the mind.

spinal stenosis—Narrowing of the lumbar spinal column that produces pressure on the nerve roots resulting in sciatica and that usually occurs in middle or old age.

SSRI—Selective serotonin reuptake inhibitor. Any of a class of antidepressants (such as fluoxetine or sertraline) that inhibit the inactivation of serotonin by blocking its reuptake by presynaptic nerve-cell endings.

steroid hormone—Any of numerous hormones (such as estrogen, testosterone, cortisone and aldosterone) with a characteristic chemical composition and formed in the body from cholesterol.

substance P—A neuropeptide that consists of 11 amino-acid residues, that is widely distributed in the brain, spinal cord and peripheral nervous system and that acts across nerve synapses to produce prolonged postsynaptic excitation.

sympathetic nervous system—The part of the autonomic nervous system that is concerned especially with preparing the body to react to situations of stress or emergency, that tends to depress secretion, decrease the tone and contractility of smooth muscle and increase heart rate.

synapse—The place at which a nervous impulse passes from one neuron to another.

systemic—Of, relating to or common to a system; affecting the entire body.

T cell—Any of several lymphocytes (such as a helper T cell) that possess highly specific cell-surface antigen receptors, and include some that control the initiation or suppression of immunity (such as by the regulation of T- and B-cell maturation and proliferation). Also called T lymphocyte.

T3—*See* **tri-iodothyronine.**

T4—*See* **thyroxine.**

TCA—*See* **tricyclic antidepressant.**

testosterone—A male hormone produced primarily by the testes or made synthetically and that is the main androgen responsible for inducing and maintaining male secondary sex characteristics.

thyrotropin—A hormone secreted by the pituitary gland that regulates the formation and secretion of thyroid hormone. Also called thyroid-stimulating hormone or thyrotropic hormone. Abbreviated TSH.

thyroxine—An iodine-containing hormone that is an amino acid produced by the thyroid gland, increases the metabolic rate and is used to treat thyroid disorders. Also called T4.

transdermal—Relating to, being or supplying a medication in a form for absorption through the skin into the bloodstream.

tricyclic antidepressant—Any of a group of antidepressant drugs (such as imipramine, amitriptyline, desipramine and nortriptyline) that contain three fused benzene rings, that potentiate the action of norepinephrine and serotonin by inhibiting their uptake by nerve endings and that do not inhibit the action of monoamine oxidase. Abbreviated TCA.

tri-iodothyronine—An iodine-containing hormone that is an amino acid derived from thyroxine and is used especially in the treatment of hypothyroidism and metabolic insufficiency. Also called liothyronine or T3.

TSH—*See* **thyrotropin.**

unsaturated fat—Fats that are from vegetable sources and are liquid at room temperature; they are good sources of essential fatty acids. (Canola, olive, corn, sunflower and safflower oils are high in unsaturated fats.)

Western blot—A blot consisting of a sheet of cellulose nitrate or nylon that contains spots of protein for identification and is used especially for the detection of antibodies.

INDEX

Improve Your Spiritual, Physical, Mental and Emotional Health

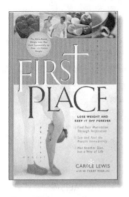

First Place
Lose Weight and Keep It Off
Carole Lewis and *Terry Whalin*
Hardcover • 216p
ISBN 08307.28635

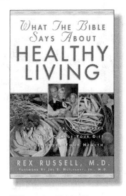

What the Bible Says About Healthy Living
Three Biblical Principles That Will Change Your Diet and Improve Your Health
Rex Russell, M. D.
Paperback • 284p
ISBN 08307.18583

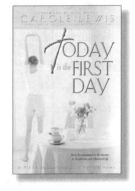

Today Is the First Day
Encouragement on the Journey to Weight Loss and a Balanced Life
Carole Lewis, General Editor
Hardcover • 386p
ISBN 08307.30656

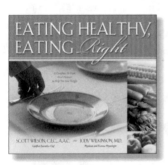

Eating Healthy, Eating Right
A Complete 16-Week Meal Planner to Help You Lose Weight
Scott Wilson, CEC, AAC
and *Jody Wilkinson,* M.D.
Hardcover • 200p
ISBN 08307.30222

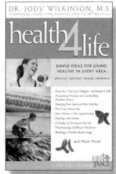

Health 4 Life
55 Simple Ideas for Living Healthy in Every Area
Jody Wilkinson, M.D.
Paperback • 240p
ISBN 08307.30516

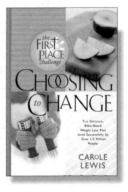

Choosing to Change
A 16-Week Challenge to Help You Reach Your Weight-Loss Goals
Carole Lewis, General Editor
Paperback • 100p
ISBN 08307.28627

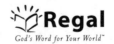